P9-BYC-936

DIABETES AND DENMARK

Edited by
Christian Binder, Torsten Deckert and Jørn Nerup

GAD PUBLISHERS

Diabetes and Denmark

Translation: Carol Bang-Christensen, except for chapters by Dr. Ørskov and Dr. Gale.
Design: Balle Grafik/Linda Balle
Reprographics and printing: Narayana Press, Gylling
ISBN: 978-87-12-04358-4

First published in Denmark in 2007

Printed in Denmark

Gad Publishers
Klosterstræde 9
1157 København K
www.gads-forlag.dk

CONTENT

PREFACE

Diabetes research in the broadest sense has been an area of special Danish strength throughout almost an entire century. Supported by a multiplicity of environments and persons, this has been an area in which institutions and enterprises have been important, but where ideas and initiatives have played a more decisive role for the results than has top-down coordinated administration.

On the occasion of Steno Diabetes Center's 75th anniversary, we have been asked to edit a book designed to give a picture of the premises, background and consequences of a number of Danish contributions to diabetes research of international standard. The essay was chosen as the genre that would allow a personal element to be combined with a specialized content. We have had sole responsibility for the choice of topics and authors. All the authors have been eyewitnesses to or directly involved in the events described. They were invited to give their personal view of their subject focusing on the interaction between the human and institutional factors they consider to be important for the results achieved.

Apart from Chapter 1, we have chosen not to be contributors even though the 75th anniversary of Steno Diabetes Center and the 50th anniversary of Hagedorn Research Institute would seem to provide a natural occasion. Instead, we have seen our role as sparring partners for the authors, who all accepted our invitation with great enthusiasm and interest. We wish to thank the authors for their exemplary cooperation.

The illustrations to the book are our responsibility. The choice of pictures has been effectively supplemented by Susanne Svendsen, MA, Dorthe Dahlsgaard Olsen, MA, and Pia Seidel, graphic designer, all from Novo Nordisk History- and Art Collection, whom we thank for their extensive efforts on behalf of the book.

We also wish to thank Steno Diabetes Center for the confidence, editorial freedom and good working conditions we have enjoyed. Furthermore, the Novo Nordisk Foundation must be thanked for a generous donation in support of the publication.

Many thanks go to Chief Physician Ebbe Eldrup, MD, DMSc, who has been a good support and who has been responsible for the actual publication process. Special thanks to course administrator Lene Krog, who with her extensive experience has made a crucial contribution to the completion of both the Danish and English manuscripts. Finally, thanks to PA Nina Meier for having taken care of many of the practical tasks.

We hope that readers will feel both enlightened and entertained and will find inspiration to search for their own answers to the questions that have been left unanswered. We also hope that the book will be read not only by health professionals specializing in diabetes but by all who are interested in optimizing the conditions for people with a chronic disease such as diabetes.

It is likewise our hope that the individual contributions may enter – nationally and internationally – into the debate concerning the development and management of both research into and treatment of a disease that burdens not only those afflicted by it but also society as a whole.

Christian Binder Torsten Deckert Jørn Nerup

WHY ...

CHRISTIAN BINDER, TORSTEN DECKERT & JØRN NERUP

WHY has Danish diabetology occupied so strong a position for so many years? There can scarcely be a simple answer to this sound and interesting question, one that foreign colleagues often ask. What is it that determines the emergence of strong artistic and scientific environments in a certain area at a certain time?

WHY did art, philosophy and the natural and health sciences flourish in Europe, in the Netherlands in particular, but also in Scandinavia in the period from the Late Renaissance and on into the Enlightenment. Just think, for instance, of names like Erasmus of Rotterdam, Rembrandt, Rubens, Descartes, Spinoza, Molière, Galileo, Newton, Roemer, Harvey, Locke, Steno and Linné. Was it a mere coincidence that these and many others appeared during this period? Or was it a consequence of the impact of the new geographical discoveries, new trade and cultural contacts with new nationalities, the general growth in prosperity and the formation of the politically more aware, more wealthy and influential middle class? And was it in fact a kind of first "globalization" that the world experienced in these years?

WHY was it under these very conditions that common sense and rationality displaced both religious belief and superstition and reduced the influence of the church on humankind and society? Was it a matter of a particularly favourable attitude to art and science among the political and economic leaders of the day and a special belief that brilliant art and original science can be purchased for money? And were there in fact massive investments in art and science in these years?

Or was it simply that the new era's new impressions and political shifts of power in a world with a new and greater openness created a climate in which the individual original thinker could freely exercise his or her talents and often in opposition to the establishment – also without having a personal background among the elite?

And WHY did art and science wither throughout the larger part of a century, for instance under the Soviet regime and what followed, and for a quarter of a century in Nazi Germany and in the following period? Was it the material circumstances in general, the closedness of society or the lack of opportunity for free intellectual life that was the cause? Or was it simply the massive exodus of intellectuals that led to the decline and the long time it took to regain the artistic and scientific levels of former times?

Many questions that require many answers. But is it not most likely that art and science will always prosper most in transparent societies that are characterized by openness, social security and balance, unimpeded international contacts, good subsidy schemes and above all room and opportunities for the individual to make use of his or her talents?

That Denmark has corresponded to this description to a varying but increasing degree in the course of the 20th century can scarcely give rise to much discussion. It can easily be documented that Danish culture and science have obtained an impressive placing in the course of the past century.

But WHY has Danish diabetology in particular placed itself so strongly? It can also be documented that this is the case. Danish diabetologists have contributed a long series of original observations and findings. Danish insulin manufacturers have been responsible for virtually all improvements in insulin preparations – often produced in mutual rivalry and competition. Through clinical trials based on their own original pathophysiological observations, Danish groups have introduced principles for treatment that can increase both longevity and quality of life with astonishing effect. Basic genetic, biochemical and immunological observations have led to important scientific changes of paradigm and have resulted in new forms of pathogenetically rooted therapy being subjected to clinical trials. Danish groups have taken initiatives for and have headed many multinational consortiums. Representatives of Danish diabetology have occupied leading posts in EASD and EFSD. All this has helped to attract substantial research funds to Denmark. Recognition in the form of a large number of international prizes – e.g. the Claude Bernard Medal and the Minkowski Prize, both of which are awarded by EASD – has been given to Danes. Only five times in a more than 60-year period has the Banting Medal, which is ADA's highest scientific distinction, been given to non-Americans. Two of these were Danish.

But of course other biomedical research fields have distinguished themselves internationally. Membrane physiology and neurophysiology are good examples. And the internationally most profiled Danish research field has undoubtedly been theoretical physics with its home base in the Niels Bohr Institute. Also Danish art and design, architecture and industry have made major impacts and evoked international attention.

WHY has this happened? It can scarcely be a matter of size. Measured on a global scale, Danish enterprises are small or medium-sized. Danish research environments – and certainly not the diabetological environments – have been much smaller in size and poorer in resources than the research institutions that they compete with at an international level. But the Danish welfare society has provided a good background by offering free education at all levels and reasonably good general conditions for research. But there has been no question of society according special advantages to the field of diabetology. Nor is there anything to indicate that Danish diabetes research has been the object of special interest on the part of private foundations and sponsors. The success of the insulin manufacturers has permitted them to use their profits and to set up foundations to support Danish academic diabetes research to a considerable degree, but not to an extent that can alone explain the success of Danish diabetes research. The diabetes hospitals and Hagedorn Research Institute have undoubtedly played an important role too. Without them, a very considerable number of doctoral dissertations and PhD theses would probably not have seen the light of day. But Danish diabetes research would nevertheless have had a strong position. Strong environments arose outside these institutions over a 50-year period in Århus, Odense, Glostrup and Copenhagen.

It is thus not so easy to identify exactly why Danish diabetology has become such a prominent field of research. At the risk of succumbing to cultivating a romanticized view of the research scientist, it is probably reasonable to point out nevertheless that, as a general feature, developments in academic and industrial diabetes research have been driven by individual researchers. Stubborn, persistent and charismatic personalities who, with different backgrounds and no doubt different motives, have pursued their own ideas through thick and thin – and have achieved significant results.

In a series of chapters, this book presents descriptions of important Danish contributions to diabetes research over a span of just under a century. All the authors have been close to events either because they were directly involved or as eyewitnesses. It is the editors' hope that readers will feel both informed and entertained, and that the individual reader will be inspired to look for answers to the many questions left unanswered in this chapter.

Present-day biomedical research – also diabetes research – is resource-demanding, multidisciplinary, often multinational and to a large extent technology driven. It produces massive quantities of data that necessitate complicated bioinformatics platforms so that we can digest and understand what we see. Great research will undoubtedly be produced in large amounts but, as is often the case, it will probably be concerned with problems that respect existing paradigms.

If anyone asks the question WHY we believe that Danish diabetes research will continue to occupy a strong position in the future, the answer will be simple. In Denmark, we probably have a touch of positive and productive anarchism. We like to see scientific paradigms fall and we have been good at making room for the individual, the controversial, the "skewed" thinker in our scientific environments. And, in the end, it may still be he or she that will radically change the direction of research, overturn the paradigms and produce the 21st century's most important contribution to Danish and international diabetes research.

FROM HAGEDORN – NORMAN JENSEN'S BLOOD GLUCOSE METHOD TO INSULIN ANALOGUES

CLAUS KÜHL

Denmark has certainly made history within the area of diabetes research and treatment; one of the reasons being that Danish diabetes researchers have been in the right place at the right time. Since the discovery of insulin in 1921, tremendous progress has been made in type 1 diabetes treatment – type 1 diabetes is henceforth referred to as "diabetes". From being an illness where only very few would survive more than a few years, diabetes has become an illness where the patient has the possibility of having a normal life expectancy and quality of life. Numerous significant breakthroughs within the area of insulin preparations and their administration stem from Denmark and can be accredited to strong, targeted diabetes research largely supported by the industry. Novo Nordisk has long conducted intensive research into diabetes and diabetes treatment and has understood the importance of good cooperation with the research environments in universities, both at home and abroad.

Hans Christian Hagedorn

Before insulin became accessible, dietary measures and physical activity were the only therapeutic options available to lower the level of glucose in the urine. In 1915, Hans Christian Hagedorn was appointed as a physician in the new hospital in Brande. He was interested in the treatment of diabetes, and examined different foodstuffs containing high levels of carbohydrates with the hope of finding some that would give only a marginal increase in the level of glucose in the urine. In Lund, Professor Bang developed a micromethod to measure the level of blood glucose that required only 0.2 ml of blood as opposed to the 10 ml formerly needed. The method was complicated and imprecise which is why Hagedorn, in cooperation with Birger Norman Jensen, a dispensing chemist at the also newly established Brande pharmacy,

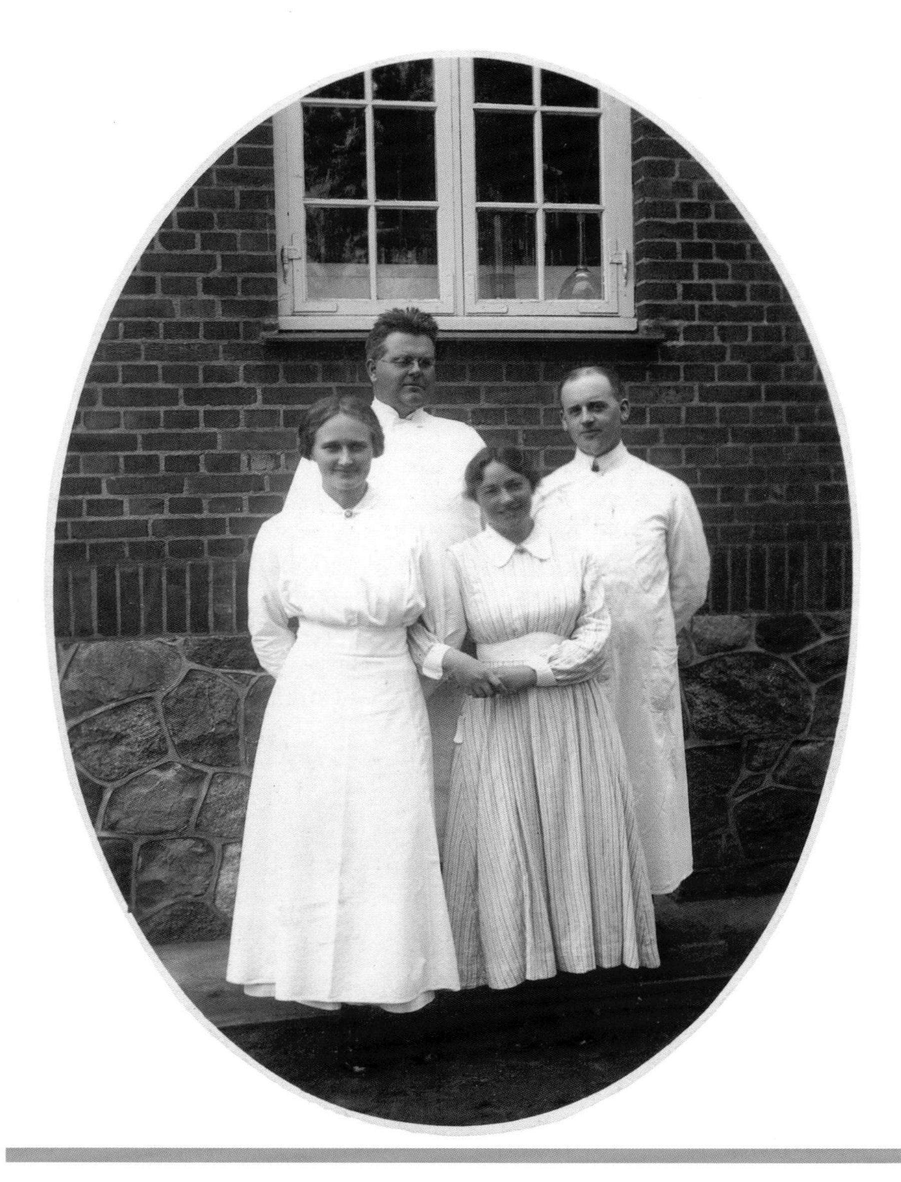

The first practical micro-method for determining blood glucose was developed in Brande in 1918. At the back: the inventors, Doctor HC Hagedorn (left) and Pharmacist Birger Norman Jensen. In front: Senior Nurse E Skovbjerg, called "Stuba", arm in arm with Hagedorn's wife Maria, called "Mitte". The building is Brande Hospital, which Hagedorn had persuaded the parish council to reopen in 1915.

improved Bang's reduction method to make it more stable and less time consuming. The method was used in Hagedorn's doctoral thesis "Blood glucose regulation in humans" [1]. It became known and employed worldwide and it was not until the 1960s that it was displaced by the enzymatic methods. The enzyme used – glucose oxidase – was discovered and further purified by Detlev Müller in August Krogh's laboratory in 1923 [2].

Hagedorn's work attracted so much attention that 1919 saw him move to Copenhagen where his work in both the scientific and clinical field gained him an increasing reputation within the area of diabetes.

August Krogh

The Danish professor August Krogh, who was awarded the Nobel Prize in 1920 in the field of physiology and medicine, was on a lecturing trip in the United States in the autumn of 1922, which is where he heard of Banting and Best' s results with insulin treatment of diabetic dogs. Encouraged by his wife, Marie Krogh, August Krogh decided to visit Professor Macleod, head of the institute in Toronto where Banting and Best had produced the world's first insulin extract from the pancreas of an ox. On 23 January 1922, the first patient had been injected with 15 ml of this extract with the fine result that the level of blood glucose dropped.

Marie Krogh, herself an MD and DMSc and also suffering from diabetes, had several patients with diabetes in her medical practice. Like her husband, she was also very interested in the new epoch-making treatment possibility. Despite the visit lasting only two days, it resulted in August Krogh leaving with both the formula and the authorisation to introduce insulin in Scandinavia. Thus, with an impressive foresight, Banting, Best and Macleod assigned the gratuitous

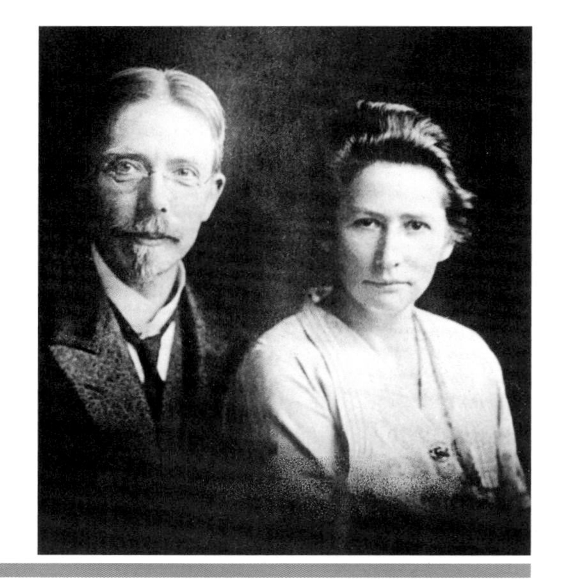

Professor August Krogh with his wife, Marie Krogh DMSc, photographed in 1920, when August Krogh was awarded the Nobel Prize in Medicine.

rights to produce insulin to August Krogh. They also assigned the rights to laboratories in other countries, provided a high ethical and scientific standard was upheld.

Nordisk Insulinlaboratorium

Krogh teamed up with Hagedorn, then a registrar of the third department of Kommunehospitalet, Copenhagen. During the winter, Hagedorn produced Denmark's first insulin in his home in Hellerup. It was dry material that needed to be dissolved immediately before injection. The first insulin injection was given in Kommunehospitalet in March 1923. The funding for the continued production of insulin came from the pharmacist August Kongsted, the owner of Leo Pharma. This is why insulins produced from 1923 by the independent institution Nordisk Insulinlaboratorium (NIL), for many years bore the name "Leo". To assist him, Hagedorn employed two brothers Harald and Thorvald Pedersen. Harald Pedersen had trained as a smith and an engineer and had been attached to Zoophysiological Laboratorium with August Krogh since 1917. Thorvald Pedersen, a qualified pharmacist, came to NIL from Dansk Sojakage Ltd. where he had been employed as a chemist.

Novo

Cooperation between Hagedorn and Thorvald Pedersen was not good. Thus, Thorvald Pedersen left NIL in 1924; out of loyalty, his brother followed. Together they began the production of insulin in the basement of a house in Frederiksberg. In 1924, the first dissolved insulin preparation, *Insulin Novo*, was introduced in Denmark. On 16 February 1925, the brothers Pedersen founded Novo Terapeutisk Laboratorium (Novo). *Insulin Novo* was sold together with a special hypodermic syringe, the *Novo Syringe*, created by Harald Pedersen. Sales of this syringe came to an end in 1944, as it was no longer possible to procure the special glass ampoules. The *Novo Syringe* meant a relief for patients. In the 1920s, they had no other option than to have up to 8 daily injections of the fast-acting insulin. It would be four decades before Novo again introduced an insulin-hypodermic syringe (*NovoPen®*).

Krogh, Hagedorn and the Pedersen brothers all exhibited an impressive pioneering spirit, determination and strong will to establish a working, consistent process to produce insulin in Denmark in a time where terms such as entrepreneur and venture capital funding were still unknown. Today, we would call these admirable pioneers entrepreneurs and the pharmacist Kongsted an early risk-taking investor.

Even though the first insulin drugs were very impure and had significant side effects, they still extended life expectancy and increased the overall quality of life for the countless diabetes patients all over the world. The need for both purer and long-acting – slow working – insulin drugs was evident. In the following decades, NIL and Novo developed and marketed insulin preparations that increasingly met these demands. Intensive research in the area of insulin chemistry and formulation coupled with intensive competition between the two companies were the driving forces behind the vastly improved insulin drugs that they produced. Both companies had competent employees who worked closely with the doctors responsible for the treatment of the patients with diabetes. Apart from the obvious commercial competition, there was also a strong, personal antagonistic relationship high up in the hierarchies. Nothing could be better than pipping the competitors to the post by being the first to introduce a new and better insulin preparation. It was two impressive, innovative companies, situated only 10 kilometres apart, which were fighting intensively to outdo each other. Rumour had it that the top management of the two companies would not use the same lift if they happened to be staying in the same hotel during scientific conferences or the likes.

Protamine insulin

The 1930s was a great decade for Danish insulin, a decade where one was taken up with finding methods to prolong insulin's effect. *Insulin + Adrenalin Novo* was marketed in 1935, but was available for only a few years. It had a long-acting period of activity, presumably due to a reduced blood flow induced by adrenalin. The first real breakthrough came in 1936, when Hagedorn, Norman Jensen and their co-workers showed that insulin could be precipitated with protamine in a neutral solution, giving a sufficiently long period of activation to make it possible to reduce the number of daily injections to 1 or 2. The new drug, *Insulin Leo Retard*, had an effect that lasted almost double that of ordinary insulin. However, the drug could last for longer periods only if it was kept in an acid solution; therefore, it had to be made neutral immediately before injection if the desired long-term effect was to be achieved.

In Joslin's textbook from 1937, the chapter on protamine insulin begins: "*Protamine insulin forms the most important development in the treatment of diabetes since insulin was discovered in 1921,...now, half a century's progress in the treatment has been completed with protamine insulin, which has opened the door to a fourth epoch that in all fairness ought to be named after its inventor in Copenhagen – Hagedorn*".

Adding small amounts of zinc salt to protamine insulin together with

Farmaceutisk Kritik af Insulin-Dommen

Man henviser til Canadieren Banting, der skænkede Menneskeheden Midlet mod Sukkersyge

Højesteretsdommen i Insulin-Sagen, der blev vundet af Dr. *Hagedorn* fra Nordisk Insulinlaboratorium, har naturligvis været stærkt drøftet i farmaceutiske Kredse, og i det sidste Nummer af Farmeceuternes Fagblad knyttes der nogle ret skarpe Kommentarer hertil. Som det vil huskes gav fem af Højesterets Dommere i Modstrid med fire Dommere Dr. Hagedorn Medhold i, at Nordisk Insulinlaboratoriums Patentrettigheder med Hensyn til Fremstilling af retarderet Insulin var blevet krænket af Terapeutisk Laboratorium Novo.

Uden Fortilfælde

Vi nærer intet Ønske om at opkaste os til Overdommere i denne Sag, skriver man i Farmaceuternes Blad, men vi har ønsket at gøre opmærksom paa, at Højesterets Afgørelse er uden Fortilfælde i dansk Patentret vedrørende Lægemidler. Vi maa desuden haabe, at denne Dom ikke maa danne Skole, for drevet ud i sin yderste Konsekvens vil dette kunne medføre, at simple Lægemiddelblandinger af en eller anden fastslaaet ny terapeutisk Virkning kan patenteres og opnaa Beskyttelse, der i betænkelig Grad nærmer

Canadieren *Banting*, skænkede Menneskeheden dette nye Lægemiddel og rundhaandet gav alle, der kunde garantere for, at Fabrikationen blev ført paa et forsvarligt Grundlag,

Retsbeskyttelse for Lægemidler?

Direktøren for Patent- og Varemærkevæsenet i Danmarks pharmaceutiske Selskab i Aftes

Højesterets Dom i Insulin-Processen mellem *Nordisk Insulin Laboratorium* og *Novo Terapeutisk Laboratorium*,

Det er muligt at faa Monopol paa Lægemidler

Anset Jurist kræver efter **Insulin-Dommen Ændringer i Patentloven**

Een Højesterets-Stemme kostede „Novo" Millioner

Selskabet skal til Nordisk Insulin-Laboratorium betale 450,000 Kr. plus 200,000 Kr. aarlig i Licensafgift for at kunne benytte Insulin-Patentet

en Licens, der nærmest er af formel Karakter, men for Eksport til Udlandet skal der betales 10 pCt. af Salgsprisen i hele Patentets Løbetid (10 Aar) — og fra Eksporttilladelsen er undtaget England og Amerika.

Desuden skal „Novo" betale Modparten 100,000 Kr. kontant og 35,000 Kr. om Aaret i 10 Aar uanset, om man fortsætter Fremstillingen af Præparatet eller ej.

Højesteretssagføreren oplyser, at „Novo" i den sidste Maaneds Tid har standset Eksporten af Insulinen, men nu genoptages den, og det vil derfor være muligt for Selskabet at beholde sine mange Medarbejdere.

Da 5 Dommere stemte for — 4 imod

Under Højesteretssagen blev Spørgsmaalet om Erstatning til Nordisk Insulin Laboratorium for Krænkelse af dets Patent ikke berørt, men antagelig maa Beløbet paa 450,000 Kr. (100,000 Kr. kontant og 35,000 om Aaret i 10 Aar), som „Novo" skal betale uanset om Præparatets Fremstilling fortsættes eller ej, skulle dække det Erstatningskrav, som Modparten mente at have Krav paa. Til dette Beløb kommer saa Licens-Afgiften, der, da „Novo"s Eksport andrager et Par Millioner Kroner

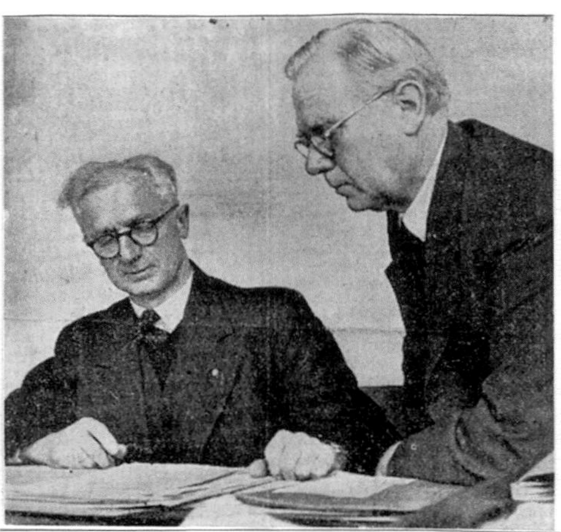

„Novo"s Ejere fotograferet i Gaar. Til venstre Fabrikejer, cand. pharm. Thorvald Pedersen, til højre Ingeniør Harald Pedersen.

Det forbudte Insulin paa Licens efter Højesterets Dom

„Novo"s Ejere har henvendt sig til Nordisk Insulin-Laboratorium for at høre Betingelserne for en

Cutting of press article on the protamine insulin suit brought by Nordisk Insulinlaboratorium against Novo in 1938: Hagedorn represented himself and conducted the case in the Supreme Court, where the verdict in 1941 went against Novo.

a surplus of protamine, created a new long-acting drug, zinc-protamine-insulin. In contrast to *Insulin Leo Retard*, this drug was ready to use and had an effect that lasted for more than 24 hours. *Zink-Protamine-Insulin Novo* was introduced on the Danish market in 1938. However, in the same year, Novo received a summons to Østre Landsret (the High Court of Eastern Denmark), as NIL was of the opinion that the production of the new Novo insulin was in breach of NIL's Danish patent covering protamine insulin. The case ended up in the Supreme Court and was decided by a majority of one vote. Novo were ruled to pay NIL 450,000 Danish Kroner and an additional annual license fee of 200,000 Danish Kroner for the duration of the patent. If cold air had existed between the two companies before, the outcome of the case added a further helping of decidedly frosty air between the two combatants.

The Danish pioneering efforts within the development of drugs continued with NPH and *Lente*®.

The Steno Memorial and Hvidøre Hospitals

NIL was the founder of Steno Memorial Hospital in 1932. The hospital quickly gained international recognition for its work with testing insulin preparations in cooperation with NIL, its clinical testing, patient education, dietary planning and systematic registration of disease progression. Novo, too, saw the great benefits of this and therefore bought Hvidøre Castle in 1937. In 1938, Hvidøre opened as Denmark's first diabetes sanatorium, and was renamed Hvidøre Hospital in 1949. In the 1970s, Steno Memorial Hospital and the somewhat smaller Hvidøre Hospital started up a joint project with Copenhagen county and Copenhagen municipality concerning check-ups and treatment of their patients with diabetes; the hospitals also accepted patients referred from many other Danish counties. Thus, the general departments of the hospitals functioned in accordance with the terms set by the Danish health authorities, whereas the extensive research activities in both places were supported by Nordisk Insulinfond and Novo respectively with additional funding from national and international foundations.

This unique set-up was visionary. It contributed to Denmark having, and still enjoying, a leading international position in diabetes research and treatment. When Novo and NIL merged to become Novo Nordisk A/S in 1989, the two hospitals were also merged to form a new, combined centre for diabetes treatment, the Steno Diabetes Center.

Significant advances were made in the scientific area during the 1960s. On the clinical front, Christian Binder showed that there are large variations in the speed at which insulin is absorbed from the injection site into the blood; a difference seen not only from patient to patient but also from day to day in individual patients. This observation, which was of significant clinical relevance, later showed to be an important part of the rationale for the development of the so-called insulin analogues.

Blood glucose meters

The 1960s also saw the development and introduction of a simple method for home monitoring of urine glucose. The method became widely used; however, it was in no way comparable to the precision and usability of the blood glucose home monitoring of the 1970s.

At the end of the 1970s, Ames introduced the *Glucometer®* which was the first appliance for home monitoring of blood glucose. The device was the size of a small shoebox, was difficult to handle and required a great care during use. Consequently, mostly laboratory technicians, doctors and nurses used the appliance. A year later, a more advanced device appeared (*Eyetone*). Since then, product development has been rapid. The present day machines are small, highly user friendly and quick and require only a few microlitres of blood. Built-in chips can remember previous measurements and even transfer these to a computer on which blood glucose profiles and much more can be generated.

Irrespective of how primitive the first appliances for home monitoring blood glucose must seem through today's eyes, they were a giant step forward and a prerequisite for the radical change in the treatment paradigm that took off in the 1980s.

For the first time, one could measure what the glucose concentration was there and then, and the patient could take the home readings to the doctor. Previously, one had had to make do with one single glucose reading from the same morning or the day before along with measuring the urine glucose. And also for the first time, patients were able to participate in the regulation of their insulin dose based on the glucose readings taken at home. The epoch of self control and own care had started.

Tight blood glucose regulation

In 1978, the French diabetologist J. Pirart [2] published the results of a long clinical study on the relationship between the quality of diabetes control and the prevalence of late complications. He showed that poor diabetes control is connected to a very high risk of developing late complications. Pirart's conclusions were supported and expanded in the large DCCT study, published in 1993 [3].

Accordingly, it became evident in the early 1980s that patients in cooperation with the treatment teams in the diabetes centres had to work hard to improve the diabetes regulation. It was no longer enough to feel well and have glucose-free urine; the target was now to achieve an average blood glucose level as close as possible to normal. In order to attain this goal, there was now access to blood glucose meters, and there was also a new analysis called HbA_{1c}, which showed the average blood glucose over the past 8-12 weeks. Preferably, the HbA_{1c} should be in the normal area (approx. 4-6 %), but it was deemed sufficient to be below 7-7.5 % in order to avoid late complications. Insulin pumps were also available. They were an excellent way to optimize treatment, but they were costly and required a certain amount of technical knowledge for proper adjustment and general maintenance, and many patients discarded the pumps for psychological reasons. On this background, the emergence of the insulin pen in the mid-1980s was an important event.

Human insulin

The beginning of the 1980s was when the Danish-manufactured highly purified insulins triumphed worldwide. Even the main competitor, American Eli Lilly (Lilly), who held a firm grip on the American market, began to feel threatened. However, Lilly had made substantial use of the Danish inventions in insulin production without having initiated equivalent development work of their own. Therefore, Lilly's drugs still contained impurities that led to high immunogenicity – the ability to create antibodies. Many American diabetes patients became aware of this; subsequently, Danish insulin preparations gained a foothold on the American insulin market. Faced with this threat, Lilly responded with an act of commercial genius. They announced that they were in the process of developing human insulin aided by a genetic engineering process invented and developed by a biotechnology corporation, Genentech. Porcine insulin differs from human insulin by having the amino acid alanin in position 30 in the B-chain, where the equivalent amino acid in human insulin is treonin. Lilly encoded a colony of the E.coli bacteria to synthesize the A-chain's 21 amino acids, while another colony was coded to synthesize the B-chain's 30 amino acids, including treonin in position 30. The two chains were subsequently merged and human insulin was thus created. However, it would take Lilly several years to optimize the new production process and to have human insulin approved by the health authorities.

The waiting time was used effectively by Novo inasmuch as Jan Markussen, in 1979 [4], had developed a process where by using enzymes it was possible to replace B_{30} in porcine insulin with treonin, thus creating semi-synthetic human insulin, and this process was quickly optimised for commercial production. Clinical trials were conducted on more than 2000 patients in more than 20 countries before Novo's human insulin was approved for marketing in 1982, which was one year earlier than the approval of Lilly's drug. In parallel, Novo developed a genetically engineered process for the production of human insulin. This process incorporated biosynthesis of a miniproinsulin molecule in baking yeast, saccharomyces cerevisiae. Later, the insulin molecule was removed and a production process for human insulin was created. NIL had not yet developed a method for the production of semi-synthetic human insulin, but was aware of the need to match Lilly and Novo. And only two years later, NIL was in a position to market similar semi-synthetic human insulin drugs.

Investigations of the insulin drugs' pharmacokinetics showed that one or two daily injections could far from match the insulin secretion 24-hour profile in healthy humans. This resulted in poor blood glucose regulation. Therefore, it was logical to improve blood glucose regulation by introducing a new form of treatment called multiple injections. It consisted of the patient injecting fast-acting insulin before each meal and long-acting insulin once every 24 hours. Multiple injections combined with frequent home monitoring of blood glucose could result in excellent blood glucose regulation among motivated patients. There was just the problem of the inconvenience of constantly having to carry insulin vials, syringes and needles, which were a necessity for all patients, children and adults alike, who were away from home for most of the day.

Insulin pens

Novo saw a commercial advantage in helping the patients by providing a solution to this problem and launched the insulin injection pen called *NovoPen®* in 1985. With *NovoPen®*, it became easy, fast and discreet for the patients to inject fast-acting insulin anywhere and anytime. NIL had chosen to focus on the development of an insulin pump, and yet again it was possible to follow in record time. One year later NIL was able to launch a pen called *Insuject®*. NIL's pen worked perfectly but was not as elegant as the *NovoPen®*, which also received a prestigious design award and was exhibited in the Museum of Modern Art in New York for several years. Denmark has remained a leader in the area of insulin pens. Today's pens are elegant and user-friendly and can have a built-in memory and be pre-loaded with sufficient insulin to cover several days' use. It was some years later that Lilly first realised the need for pens, presumably because the domestic American market was far behind that of Europe concerning modern insulin treatment and self care.

Insulin analogues

But even with multiple injections, it was a problem that the fast-acting insulin did not take effect until 30 to 60 minutes after the injection, and that the duration of the long-acting insulin, which was administered at bedtime, was often too short to effectively cover a whole night's insulin need. In Novo, Jens Brange and his co-workers [5] had succeeded in producing insulin drugs where the insulin could be found in monomer form as opposed to the known fast-acting drugs where insulin was found as hexamers, i.e., in groups of 6 insulin molecules. When insulin in hexamer form is injected, each hexamer must first be changed to at least dimer form before the insulin can be absorbed into the bloodstream. This change takes time, which is why the effect on blood glucose is not seen until 30 to 60 minutes later. Novo's first monomer insulin, X10, showed to have precisely this desirable characteristic in clinical trials. The trial had to be stopped when toxicology tests in animals showed a slight risk of developing cancer, and it was therefore necessary to reassess the development. In the meantime, Lilly had produced a monomer insulin, *Humalog®*, by switching the last two amino acids in the B-chain. This drug was on the market in 1996, whereas Novo Nordisk's first monomer insulin, *NovoRapid®*, was launched in 1999.

Another research group in Novo Nordisk, headed by Jan Markussen [6], was working on the solution for two clinically important problems with conventional long-acting insulin: the large variation in the absorption speed and the too short period of action. As Brange, Markussen also employed gene technology to produce variants (analogues) of the insulin molecule that were expected to have the desired characteristics. And just as Brange had been overtaken by Lilly in the monomer insulin area, Markussen and Novo Nordisk had to see themselves overtaken by Hoechst (later Sanofi Aventis), who came first with a long-acting insulin analogue called glargine (*Lantus®*) in 2000. Novo Nordisk's new long-acting insulin analogue, detemir (*Levemir®*), was not introduced before 2004.

Fast-acting and long-acting insulin analogues and insulin pens or pumps should, in theory, make it possible to perfect blood glucose regulation in all patients who have access to these treatment advances. While controlled studies of intensified treatment have shown that this theory can be put into practice, it has, unfortunately, also been shown that the regulation among the majority of patients deteriorates shortly after the end of the controlled study. The explanation for this is probably that the interest and attention from the treatment team has a highly motivating effect on the patients while the study is ongoing. A follow-up study of the patients who had achieved good metabolic regulation in the 9 years where they participated in the DCCT study [3] showed that most were now more poorly regulated. Something similar is observed in women with diabetes who wish to conceive. These women know that good diabetes regulation is absolutely essential for an uncomplicated pregnancy for both mother and foetus. This knowledge is incredibly motivating and by far, most women achieve excellent diabetes regulation both before and during the pregnancy. However, after giving birth, the picture changes; motivation seems to slide down the list of priorities for a new mother, leading to a worsening in diabetes regulation.

Therefore, access to insulin analogues, pens and pumps is not enough. The motivation to achieve and maintain good regulation must also be there. Patients who are motivated have shown they can achieve excellent diabetes control with conventional human insulin delivered several times a day, based on frequent home-monitored blood glucose values.

Novo Nordisk A/S

The introduction of gene technology and insulin analogues demanded not only a tremendous research effort but also very significant investment in new production facilities. There was therefore good reason for the management of NIL and Novo to make the decision that, in retrospect, they should have made years earlier. In 1989, they buried the hatchet and merged the two companies to Novo Nordisk A/S. Denmark thereby maintained a leading position within the insulin area, a position further consolidated after the merger. Those who feared the ability to compete would disappear when the neighbouring company was no longer there to be interfered with and preferably beaten on the finishing line were proven wrong. Sharp competition from Lilly and Sanofi Aventis has shown to be more than enough to keep Novo Nordisk at the forefront as regards research and product development within the insulin area.

The future

It is likely correct that human insulin is a perfect insulin, developed over thousands of years through evolution, but nature could not foresee that human insulin would be administered subcutaneously – under the skin – to humans with diabetes. Subcutaneous insulin does not go directly to the liver as opposed to insulin released from the pancreas. It therefore takes longer to take effect, but this situation is seemingly successfully balanced by the fast-acting insulin analogues. Neither did nature foresee that humans with diabetes also are in need of insulin with a long period of activation – this is where the long-acting insulin analogues play their part. Even the best long-acting human insulin drugs cannot match the analogues as regards their action profile. Should we one day reach the point where insulin can be administered safely and intraportally, human insulin must become the insulin of choice.

And what will the future then bring? The ultimate aim is, obviously, to eliminate the diabetes disease, but when will this happen? Until that time, there will be a need for still better insulin preparations and methods to administer insulin. Denmark has played a very prominent role in all this development and there is nothing that indicates that this role will diminish over the next 85 years.

REFERENCES

1. *Hagedorn HC. Blodsukkerregulationen hos mennesket. Disputats. Københavns Universitet 1921*
2. *Pirart J. Diabetes mellitus and its degenerative complications: a prospective study of 4.400 patients observed between 1947 and 1973 (in three parts). Diabete Metab 1977;3:97-107; 173-82; 245-56*
3. *The Diabetes Control and Complications Trial Research Group. The effect of intensive treatment of diabetes on the development and progression of long-term complications in insulin-dependant diabetes mellitus. N Engl J Med 1993;329:977-86*
4. *Markussen J. US Patent 4343898. 1980*
5. *Brange J, Owens D, Kang S, Vølund A. Monomeric insulins and their experimental and clinical implications. Diabetes Care 1990;13:923-54*
6. *Kurtzhals P, Havelund S, Jonassen I, Kiehr B, Larsen UD, Ribel U, Markussen J. Albumin binding of insulins acylated with fatty acids: characterization of the ligand-protein interaction and correlation between binding affinity and timing of the insulin effect in vivo. Biochem J 1995;312:725-31*

INSULIN: PURE, PURER, PUREST

KLAVS H JØRGENSEN & OLE O ANDERSEN

The road towards pure insulin

Novo Nordisk has had a decisive influence on insulin treatment with its more than 80 years of experience in purifying insulin and in the development and production of insulin preparations. As described in Chapter 2, Professor August Krogh obtained authorization to produce insulin in Denmark in 1922. Together with Dr Hans Christian Hagedorn, he founded Nordisk Insulinlaboratorium (NIL) in 1923. In 1925, a former employee Thorvald Pedersen and his brother Harald formed a competing insulin company, Novo Terapeutisk Laboratorium (Novo) [1, 2]. In 1989, the two enterprises merged as Novo Nordisk A/S.

The strong competition between the two enterprises seems to have been more beneficial than harmful. Both sought to produce insulin of high quality and under controlled conditions. Here it should be mentioned that a large proportion of the staff were dairymen, who during their training had learnt to work with great respect for cleanliness and good hygiene. The dry insulin – the base material for formulating preparations – was from the start amorphous. Insulin had already been crystallized by Abel in 1926, but his method did not reproduce well. In 1934, Scott showed that crystallization required the presence of zinc or other metals, and it was only then that crystallization could be introduced as a supplementary stage in insulin production. The biological potency of dry insulin, expressed in number of units per mg, was measured in relation to the potency of an international standard in the form of a selected dry insulin with a number of international units per mg determined by the fall in blood glucose after injection in rabbits, or determined by the frequency of convulsions as a consequence of low blood glucose after injection in mice. The biological potency of the first amorphous International Standard from 1923 was 8 IU (International Units) per mg, which shows that the first insulin produced was very impure when one considers that the potency of the purest insulin produced from the mid-1970s was 27–28 IU/mg, depending on the water and salt content of the dry insulin. In time, as production was systematized, the purity of the insulin was enhanced, so that the potency of the amorphous final product rose to close on 18 IU per mg. The Second International Standard from 1935 was produced from once crystallized insulin and had a biological potency of 22 IU/mg. Fast-acting preparations of dissolved insulin were slightly acid, because the presence of a small content of protein-degrading enzymes rendered dissolved neutral insulin unstable. The slower-acting *protamine insulin* discovered in NIL by Hagedorn and Norman Jensen in 1936 had stability problems. Shortly afterwards, Scott and Fisher in Toronto using crystallized insulin as base material created the so-called *zinc protamine insulin* (ZPI), a ready-to-use, stable, neutral, amorphous preparation with a longer-lasting effect [1, 2].

The insulin becomes purer

In 1945, a new crystallization method invented by Karl Petersen was introduced in Novo's production. The previously used phosphate buffer was replaced by a citrate buffer. The citrate method gave a quicker and more reliable crystallization with a better yield than formerly and in addition proved to give a purer insulin. Since the start of insulin treatments, an immediate but brief increase in blood glucose had been noted before the decrease set in after injection. Already in 1923, it was assumed that the effect was due to pollution by a hormone, the so-called hyperglycaemic factor (glucagon), which had been prepared from a pancreatic extract. However, citrate-crystallized insulin led to no increase in blood glucose; nor, indeed, could glucagon be shown in citrate-crystallized insulin using the methods of that time [2]. By optimizing purification prior to crystallization, NIL had achieved a corresponding improvement in the purity of the insulin, so that as early as 1946 Danish insulin preparations from both NIL and Novo were glucagon-free [1].

In 1947, on the basis of an invention by Krayenbühl and Rosenberg, NIL began to market a new long-acting insulin preparation, NPH, a stable, neutral crystalline preparation consisting of zinc, insulin and protamine, in which the protamine content was substantially lower than that in ZPI-insulin. This made it possible to mix fast-acting insulin without disturbing the effect profile of either of the two components [1]. There was at this time much confusion concerning the slow-acting insulin preparations, and a major comparative study was therefore conducted in the USA, in which NIL's new preparation was designated NPH (Neutral Protamine Hagedorn). The study turned out in favour of NPH, which became "The drug of choice" recommended by leading diabetologists from, among other institutions, the Joslin and Mayo Clinics.

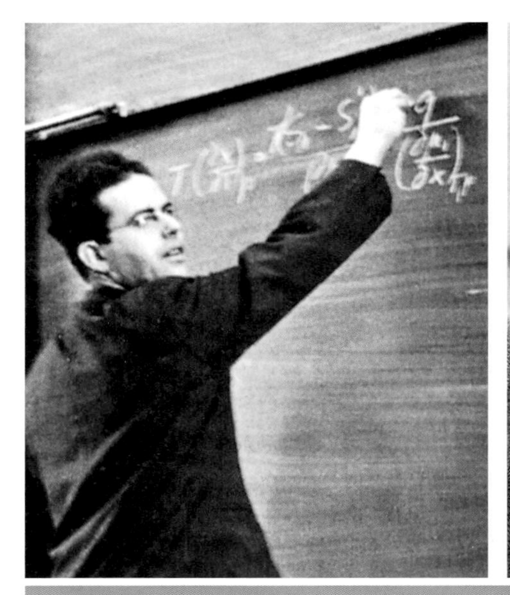

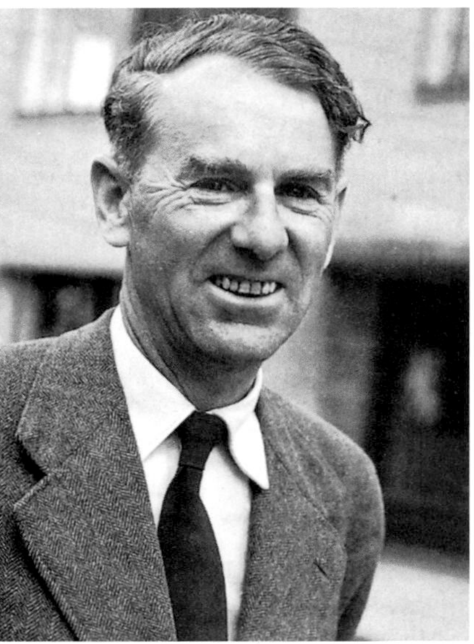

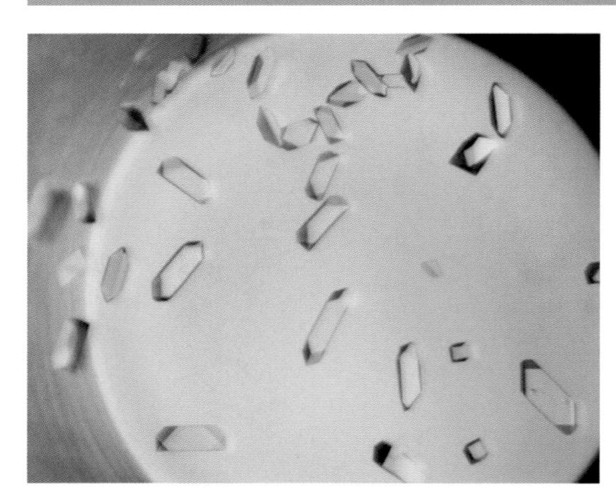

Charles Krayenbühl and Thomas Rosenberg (at the blackboard) from Nordisk Insulinlaboratorium discovered protamine insulin's crystallization ability (microphoto) in 1943. Like NPH insulin, protamine insulin is probably still the most used long-acting insulin preparation in the world.

Lente® preparations, invented by Hallas Møller, Karl Petersen and Jørgen Schlichtkrull and marketed in 1953, were Novo's response to NPH. The *Lente®* preparations, which did not contain protamine, consisted of *Ultralente®*, a stable, neutral zinc suspension of sharp-edged, rhomboedric bovine insulin crystals with a long-acting effect, and *Semilente®*, a stable, neutral zinc suspension of amorphous porcine insulin with a short-acting effect. A stable mixture, *Lente®*, of 70 % *Ultralente®* and 30 % *Semilente®*, had a good biphasic effect and was widely used. [2-4].

Citrate crystals from porcine insulin were sharp as opposed to those from bovine insulin. For use in the formulation of *Ultralente*®, Schlichtkrull found that bovine insulin too, obtained a perfectly sharp, rhomboedric form, if the crystallization took place in a highly salty acetate buffer with a certain zinc content at pH 5.5 [3, 4].

Repeated acetate crystallizations of initially citrate-crystallized insulin were introduced in Novo's insulin procedures for the production of the *Lente*® preparations. Recrystallization gave increased purity. The Fourth International Standard from 1958, produced from recrystallized insulin, exhibited a biological potency of 25 IU/mg.

Schlichtkrull subsequently found that it was possible to produce a stable, neutrally dissolved injection preparation from porcine insulin, called *Actrapid*®, if after the acetate crystallizations of porcine insulin the zinc content was reduced by finishing with a citrate crystallization. This was the first time that anything of this kind had succeeded. It had to mean that the new crystallization method had reduced the effect from pollution of the insulin by protein-degrading enzymes to an insignificant level. *Actrapid*®, which was put on the market in 1961, proved to have a quicker onset effect and caused less tissue irritation than acid-dissolved preparations [2, 4]. This made the preparation suitable as the fast-acting part of the intensified insulin treatment introduced later.

Parallel with *Actrapid*®, a biphasic preparation called *Rapitard*® was marketed. This was a biphasically-acting preparation consisting of ¼ dissolved, fast-acting porcine insulin and ¾ in suspension of slow-acting bovine insulin crystals with the same form as *Ultralente*®, but with lower zinc content [2, 4].

The purest insulin

The development towards the purest insulin is based on a number of different scientific advances in the 1950s, 1960s and 1970s.

In 1955, a group around Sanger in Cambridge succeeded in identifying the primary structures of bovine and porcine insulin. The insulin molecule is made up of an A-chain consisting of 21 amino acids and a B-chain consisting of 30 amino acids. The chains are tied together by two sulphur bridges, and in the A-chain, there is one internal sulphur bridge. The B-chains are identical in the two insulins, while there are different amino acids in positions A8 and A10. The molecular weights could be calculated as 5778 for porcine insulin and 5734 for bovine insulin [4]. Porcine insulin differs only by one amino acid in position B30 from human insulin, the structure of which was elucidated by Nicol and Smith in 1960.

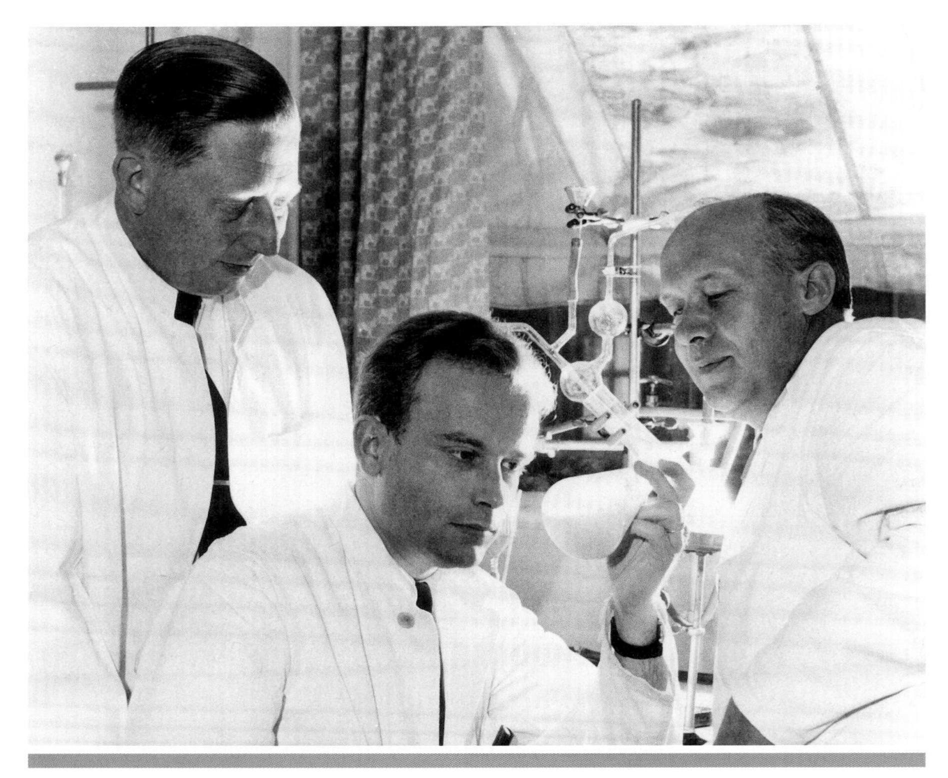

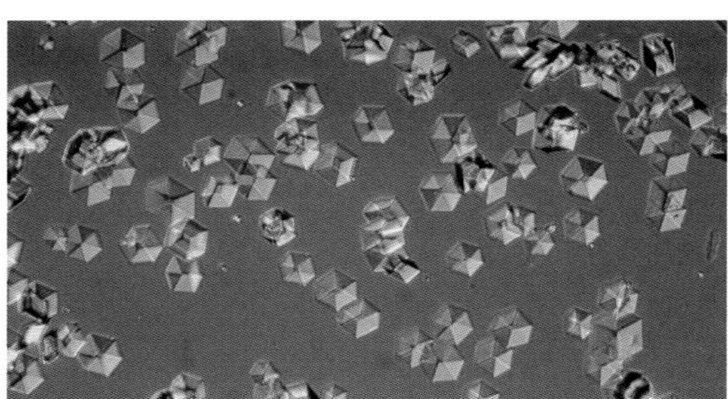

The team at Novo behind the world's purest insulin preparations. From the left: Knud Hallas-Møller, Jørgen Schlichtkrull and Karl Pedersen with microphoto of Lente® insulin crystals.

The presence of insulin-degrading factors in plasma in patients treated with insulin had been demonstrated as early as 1928, but it was not until 1956 that the Americans Berson and Yalow succeeded in documenting that insulin therapy led to the formation of insulin-binding antibodies belonging to the globulin fraction in plasma. Of the 25 diabetes patients investigated, who had been treated with insulin for more than three months, all had insulin-binding antibodies in their serum [5].

Already in 1922, Joslin had described localized allergic dermal reactions at injection sites after injection with insulin. Allergic reactions in connection with insulin therapy were frequent, particularly in the USA, from where at the start of the 1960s, there were reports of localized reactions in up to 25-50 % of patients. Universal reactions occurred more rarely, but were encountered in 1-2 % of patients. In Denmark, allergic reactions to insulin have been extremely rare. Thus, Deckert found in 1964 [6] that at Steno Memorial Hospital only 1-2 occurrences of universal reactions had been registered since the mid-1950s. Deckert concluded that impurities in the insulin preparations must have caused the insulin allergy.

It was, however, the prevailing view that the insulin molecule was in itself immunogenic, that is to say responsible for the formation of circulating insulin antibodies. This was supported by Deckert in his doctoral thesis "Insulin Antibodies" from 1964 [6]. His studies showed that highly purified porcine insulin produced by continuous electrophoresis was only minimally immunogenic in rabbits, and that certain impurities gave rise to the formation of antibodies that were different from insulin antibodies. Together with Brunfeldt, he further showed that insulin antibody formation was intensified when the insulin preparations were impure. This might be due to a kind of adjuvant effect, i.e., that the impurities supported the formation of insulin antibodies.

In the course of the 1960s, it was surprisingly demonstrated with the help of a new method of analysis that insulin – also even if it had been purified via repeated crystallizations – contained small quantities of a range of impurities. These impurities were in particular made visible by Mirsky and Kawamura in 1964 via discontinuous electrophoresis, which separates proteins according to charge and to some degree also according to size [4].

In a lecture in 1967, Steiner and Oyer reported that the synthesis of insulin in human beta-cells occurs via a precursory stage (prohormone), called proinsulin [7]. This was the first prohormone to be discovered. Steiner's lecture made a strong impression on the audience thanks to its technically elegant and convincing presentation. It was sensed that a groundbreaking discovery had been made public, even though the lecture was delivered in a relaxed and slightly understated manner.

In 1968, Steiner et al demonstrated through gel filtration that crystalline bovine insulin contained a minor impurity fraction, the b-component, with higher molecular weight than the c-component, which contained the actual insulin. By separating the b-component, it was possible to isolate, among other things, a component that could be identified as proinsulin, which could be converted into insulin with the aid of enzymes. The structure of porcine insulin was published by Chance et al in 1969 and 1970. The molecular weight is approx. 9000, against insulin's approx. 6000. It appears that insulin's two chains are linked via a peptide chain containing the so-called C-peptide. The amino acid sequence of the C-peptide varies considerably from species to species.

The occurrence of several impurities, not least proinsulin, gave the impetus to attempts to further purify insulin. In this respect, Denmark once again came to play a significant role via the Novo Research Institute (NRI) and NIL.

NRI was established in 1964 within the framework of Novo and with Jørgen Schlichtkrull as head of institute in recognition of his scientific work in connection with the *Lente®* preparations. NRI was given the freedom to carry out basic research in the field of diabetes in the widest sense. Schlichtkrull's sister had insulin-dependent diabetes, and shortly after the establishment of NRI, his daughter was also diagnosed with this disease. This was a cause of great concern for him but it was also a motivating factor in his work. Schlichtkrull was highly respected by his colleagues at home and abroad, and with his stringency, his high demands for quality and his openness to discussion, he was of enormous importance as a mentor for a large number of researchers. His sense of irony and black humour did, however, often lead him into conflicts.

After the discovery of proinsulin, research into the immunogenicity of insulin – its ability to form antibodies – and the clinical significance of this phenomenon was intensified both at NRI and at Steno Memorial Hospital. The work at NRI took its starting point in gel filtration of once-crystallized porcine and bovine insulin. The impurities were divided into three components, each of which was shown to be heterogeneous via discontinuous electrophoresis: the a-component, consisting of high-molecular-weight proteins and containing a small amount of incorporated immunoreactive insulin; the b-component, consisting of polypeptides with molecular weights between 8000 and 12,000, including proinsulin and partially degraded products from it and a so-called covalent insulin dimer; and the c-component with a molecular weight of around 6000 (about the same as for insulin), including insulin, mono- and diarginine insulin, ethylesters of insulin and desamidoinsulins. The last two groups are formed during the production process. Together, the impurities constituted between 5 and 10 % of the insulin.

On this background, Schlichtkrull got the idea that it was the impurities in conventional insulin that were in themselves responsible for the formation of the circulating insulin antibodies, and that pure insulin itself was not immunogenic. The idea was tested in animal experiments in a collaboration between staff from NRI and Novo's insulin laboratories. The various insulin impurities were isolated from crystalline insulin. After subcutaneous injection of 40 micrograms of the fraction in rabbits three times weekly, the immunogenicity was analysed by measuring the concentration of insulin antibodies in blood taken in the course of the following 100 days. The results were compared with the corresponding results after injection of recrystallized insulin and of insulin that had essentially been freed of impurities.

The results accorded with Deckert's studies from 1964 in the sense that the impurities in the insulin were of significant importance for the formation of circulating antibodies, and the pure insulin itself was immunogenic only to a small degree, but on the other hand, the results did not agree with Deckert's supposed causal relationship, which is described above.

The high molecular a-component was most immunogenic in regard to the formation of insulin antibodies. After this, came the b-component, proinsulin, recrystallized insulin and finally impurities from the c-component. Impurities from bovine insulin proved on the whole to be more immunogenic than the corresponding impurities from porcine insulin, while the pure porcine insulin and the pure bovine insulin that had been produced using the method described below were both non-immunogenic in the chosen animal model [8]. Shortly after, the findings were presented in a lecture in 1969.

The idea was tested on patients with newly diagnosed diabetes treated with insulin that was pure according to the most sensitive analysis techniques of the day, discontinuous electrophoresis and gel filtration. This pure insulin was designated *monocomponent insulin* or simply *MC insulin*.

For the manufacturing of large quantities of *MC insulin*, Jørgensen developed a new particularly production-efficient purification method based on column chromatographic anion exchange in an ethanolic medium [8, 9]. The method was presented in a lecture in 1970. Patent applications were filed for both an injectible preparation consisting of *MC insulin* and the purification method in 1969.

The first clinical trial of *MC insulin* at Hvidøre Hospital showed that in the patients who were treated from the start with porcine *MC insulin*, formulated as *Lente®* – called *Monotard®* – the insulin antibody level after approx. one year's treatment was too low to be measured in the majority of the patients and very low in the remainder. In parallel trials, *Lente®* preparations based on repeatedly crystallized bovine and porcine insulin, or porcine insulin alone, proved markedly immunogenic – bovine insulin most so. The results, which fully met the expectations from the animal trials, were ready in 1970 [8, 9]. The publications in the beginning of the 1970s evoked considerable interest and were the prelude to a number of clinical trials in Europe, which confirmed that the formation of circulating insulin antibodies could be avoided or reduced in patients with insulin-dependent diabetes. It appeared that in the course of some months, the change from conventional insulin to porcine *MC insulin* led to a decreasing need for insulin. An unexpected advantage was that lipoatrophy – loss of fatty tissue at the injection sites, a side-effect that had previously been unavoidable for certain patients – could be eliminated via the switch. Porcine *MC insulin* preparations in the form of *Actrapid®*, *Semilente®* and *Lente®* (*Monotard®*) were put on the market in 1973-74.

In 1973, Ortved Andersen showed in studies at Steno Memorial Hospital that patients treated with conventional insulin preparations containing 1-2 % proinsulin formed specific proinsulin antibodies that reacted only with species-specific proinsulin and partially degraded proinsulin, but not with C-peptide or insulin [10].

Later studies at NRI showed that antibodies against parts of impurities that did not include the insulin molecule, for instance part of the a-component and other pancreatic polypeptides, demonstrated in patients treated with Novo's conventional preparations, were absent in patients treated with *MC insulin* [4, 9].

NIL followed close on Novo's heels with the development of highly purified porcine insulin, which in the form of NPH and neutrally dissolved insulin was put on the market in 1974 with the designation RI (*rare immunogenum*). The same year, Deckert and colleagues published [11] a clinical study of highly purified porcine NPH at Steno Memorial Hospital. The findings confirmed that the formation of circulating insulin antibodies could be avoided or reduced in patients treated with the highly purified insulin, which also led to a reduction of the insulin dose and lipoatrophy.

In 1974, Heding et al at NRI developed radioimmunoassays for bovine and porcine C-peptide [12]. This made it possible to determine the content of specifically proinsulin-like

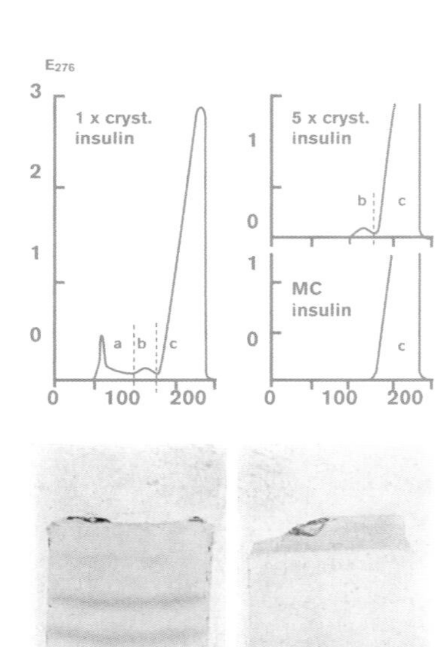

Top: a graphic representation of gel filtering of insulin after 1st and 5th crystallizations and after purification to MC insulin. Below: electrophoretic fractioning of insulin after the first crystallization and after further purification to MC insulin. (Data from the author).

immunoreactive components (PLI) in insulin preparations. The PLI content was determined at 1–2 % corresponding to 10,000–20,000 ppm (parts per million) in conventional, repeatedly crystallized insulin, and approx. 500 ppm in *MC insulin*, which was also the level in NIL's highly purified insulin. With the object of further reducing PLI, a new adsorption chromatographic purification method was developed and introduced in production. In combination with the aforementioned purification method based on anion exchange chromatography, *MC insulin* with a PLI content < 1 ppm was attained. Additionally, the content of other pancreatic polypeptides that could be determined via specific radioimmunoassay was reduced significantly to < 1 ppm [13].

In 1977, twice chromatographed bovine *MC insulin* was put on the market, so that the entire range of Novo's insulin preparations were on offer in *MC* quality. Bovine *MC insulin* was considerably less immunogenic than conventional bovine insulin in patients, but showed to be more immunogenic than porcine *MC insulin*. The presumption that the insulin impurities caused the formation of circulating antibodies had proved correct, although they did not appear to be the sole cause. The species of the pure insulin could not be entirely disregarded. The obvious clinical benefits and the intense publication and promotional activities made *MC insulin* a major financial success [2].

Comprehensive biological potency determinations using the mouse convulsions method carried out by Pingel et al in 1982 [14] showed that *MC insulin*'s biological potency is 29 IU/mg without water and salt and, as mentioned above, 27–28 IU/mg for ordinary monocomponent dry insulin depending on the water and salt content.

The experience gained on the way towards the purest porcine and bovine insulin has been of crucial importance for the purity attained for the subsequently marketed preparations of human insulin and insulin analogues.

In the course of the 1970s, a number of studies were able to confirm that highly purified or *MC insulin* was effective in treatment of insulin allergy, and today it is generally recognized that it is impurities in the insulin preparations that have been responsible for allergic manifestations.

Whether insulin in itself is immunogenic, as formerly supposed, is doubtful and is at all events open to discussion. According to current view, a molecule must be of a certain size for it to be able in itself to give rise to antibody formation. In the light of the non-existent or very low immunogenicity of *MC insulin* and highly purified insulin, it is our view that insulin as such scarcely fulfils these conditions.

It is characteristic of smaller molecules, socalled haptens, that they are not in themselves immunogenic, but can be made immunogenic by, for instance, covalent bonding to polypeptides. This seems precisely to be the case for insulin impurities such as a-component, which contains non-insulin polypeptide-covalently bonded to immunoreactive insulin, and for animal proinsulin, which besides the insulin molecule contains a polypeptide chain with a sequence that deviates from the corresponding chain in human proinsulin.

Even though insulin in itself is thus unlikely to be immunogenic, the presence of insulin in hexamer form in neutral solutions, or even in corpuscular forms in suspensions, can well be imagined to make the non-immunogenic insulin molecule immunogenic. The results from treatment with *MC-Lente®* preparations (sometimes in combination with *MC-Actrapid®*) and highly purified NPH-insulin do not, however, indicate that such a mechanism is of major significance.

Up to the beginning of the 1970s, insulin resistance (insulin need > 200 IU/day) in patients with type 1 diabetes was found to occur with a frequency of 3 % in a number of countries. Deckert was, however, able to discover only 2 cases in Denmark in the period 1950-1964. In a later survey, he found only 1 case among 1006 patients with type 1 diabetes. The change to treatment with highly purified insulin preparations has proved to be effective in the treatment of insulin resistance. This indicates that insulin resistance in patients with type 1 diabetes has been conditional on antibodies caused by impurities in the insulin preparations.

Several studies from the 1970s showed lower insulin needs in non-insulin resistant patients treated with highly purified insulins as well as correlation between insulin need and the titre of antibodies and parallel fall in insulin need and antibody titre when converted from recrystallized to highly purified insulins [10]. Partial or complete remission or honeymoon occurs early in the course in about 40 % of patients with type 1 diabetes with a declining need of insulin lasting for weeks up to many months. Shorter remission periods were observed in patients who developed antibodies [10].

Insulin antibodies may also neutralise the effect of endogenous insulin, which be of importance for patients who temporarily may be in need of insulin treatment such as women with gestational diabetes [10].

Severe late-diabetic eye and kidney complications are especially seen in patients with longer-lasting type 1 diabetes. Some studies have indicated that patients with a special tissue type could develop particularly high contents of insulin antibodies, possibly with special – e.g. strongly binding or complex-forming – properties. It has been demonstrated that such patients had more frequent occurrences of severe eye changes and early onset of kidney effects. Despite the tendency of a number of studies, it must still be regarded as an unresolved question whether insulin antibodies can provoke the development of severe late-diabetic complications.

REFERENCES

1. *Deckert T. Dr. Med. H.C. Hagedorn og det danske insulin-eventyr. Herning: Poul Christensens Publisher, 1998*
2. *Richter-Friis H. Livet på Novo. Copenhagen: Gyldendal, 1991*
3. *Schlichtkrull J. Insulin crystals. Chemical and biological studies on insulin crystals and insulin zinc suspensions. Doctoral thesis. Copenhagen: Ejnar Munksgaard Publisher, 1958*
4. *Brange J, Skelbaek-Pedersen B, Langkjaer L, Damgaard U, Ege H, Havelund S, Heding LG, Jørgensen KH, Lykkeberg J, Markussen J, Pingel M, Rasmussen E. Galenics of insulin: The physico-chemical and pharmaceutical of insulin and insulin preparations. Berlin Heidelberg New York London Paris Tokyo: Springer-Verlag, 1987*
5. *Berson SA, Yalow RS, Bauman A, Rothschild MA, Newerly K. Insulin-I^{131} metabolism in human subjects: Demonstration of insulin binding globulin in the circulation of insulin-treated subjects. J Clin Invest 1956;35:170-90*
6. *Deckert T. Insulin Antibodies. Doctoral thesis. Copenhagen: Ejnar Munksgaard Publisher, 1964*
7. *Steiner DF, Oyer PE. The biosynthesis of insulin and a probable precursor of insulin by a human islet cell adenoma. Proc Nat Acad Sci US 1967;57:473-80*
8. *Schlichtkrull J, Brange J, Christiansen AaH, Hallund O, Heding LG, Jørgensen KH. Clinical aspects of insulin-antigenicity. Diabetes 1972;21(Suppl 2):649-56*
9. *Schlichtkrull J, Brange J, Christiansen AaH, Hallund O, Heding LG, Jørgensen KH, Rasmussen SM, Sørensen E, Vølund Aa. Monocomponent insulin and its clinical implications. Horm Metab Res 1974;5(Suppl.Ser.):134-43*
10. *Andersen OO. Anti-insulin-antistoffer: Faktorer af betydning for deres dannelse. Anti-insulin-antistoffers kliniske betydning. Doctoral thesis. Copenhagen Århus Odense: Publisher: FADL, 1977*
11. *Deckert T, Andersen OO, Poulsen JE. The clinical significance of highly purified pig- insulin preparations. Diabetology 1974;10:703-8*
12. *Heding LG, Larsen UD, Markussen J, Jørgensen KH, Hallund O. Radioimmunoassays for human, pork and ox C-peptides and related substances. Horm Metab Res 1974;5(Suppl.Ser):40-4*
13. *Jørgensen KH, Hallund O, Heding LG, Tronier B, Falholt K, Damgaard U, Thim L, Brange J. Estimation of insulin purity in light of developments in analytical methods. In: Gueriguian JL, Bransome ED, Outschoorn AS, eds. Hormone Drugs. United States Pharmacopeial Convention, Rockville, Maryland, 1982:139-47*
14. *Pingel M, Vølund Aa, Sørensen E, Sørensen AR. Assessment of insulin potency by chemical and biological methods. In: Gueriguian JL, Bransome ED, Outschoorn AS, eds. Hormone Drugs. United States Pharmacopeial Convention, Rockville, Maryland, 1982: 200-7*

INTENSIFIED TREATMENT OF PATIENTS WITH TYPE 1 AND TYPE 2 DIABETES

STEN MADSBAD

The major technological breakthroughs in the treatment of type 1 diabetes

At the end of the 1970s and in the beginning of the 1980s, came the major breakthroughs: HbA_{1c} became a routine measurement, home measurement of blood glucose became common, and the pen system was introduced along with therapy team supported self-care. Treatment with insulin pumps and pancreas transplantation became experimental treatments.

Multiple injections with quick-acting insulin before each main meal and NPH insulin at bedtime were introduced for patients with type 1 diabetes. The experience from the introduction of multiple injections still holds: the change from twice-daily insulin with a combination of quick-acting and NPH insulin to multiple injections led to only a slight improvement in HbA_{1c}, which had disappeared after 6–12 months' treatment. The conclusion is that if the degree of glycaemia regulation is to be improved, the insulin regime cannot stand alone, but must be combined with ongoing adjustments based on home measurement of blood glucose, planned intake of carbohydrates, physical activity and experience-based algorithms worked out together with the patient.

Development and clinical use of insulin pumps

At the end of the 1970s and in the beginning of the 1980s, there was focus on how a more physiological insulin profile could be attained. The "artificial pancreas", which infused insulin intravenously, made it possible to normalise the concentration of blood glucose over a shorter period in type 1 patients. Insight was also obtained into what insulin profile in the peripheric blood was most optimal in order to achieve normoglycaemia.

Insulin pumps became an important research tool for investigating the

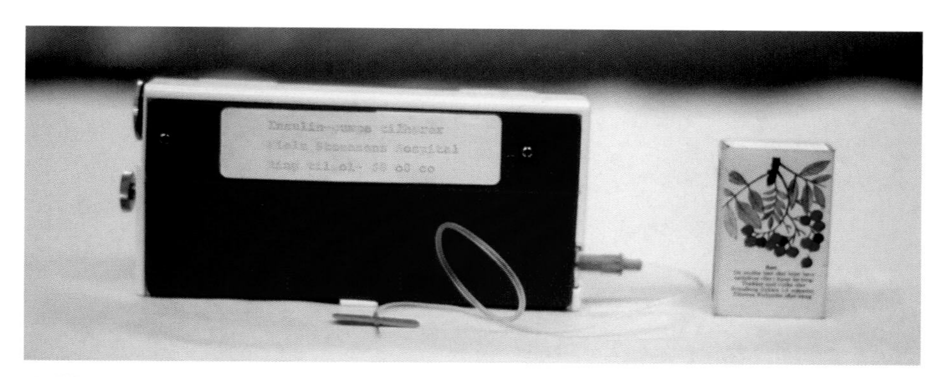

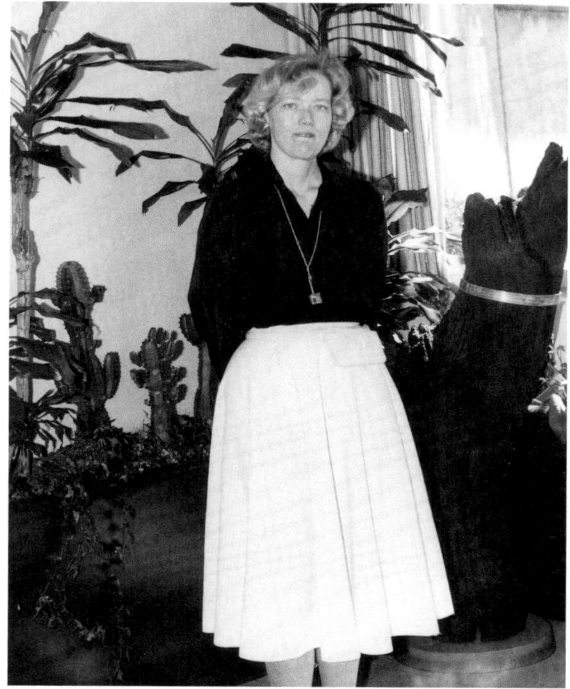

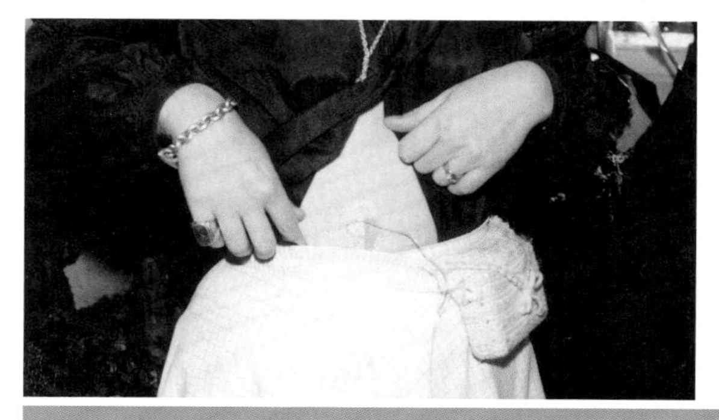

Patient with the first portable insulin pump (Mill Hill 1980) concealed in a small homemade bag in the belt. Insulin was subcutaneously administered through a thin catheter in the skin of the stomach.

importance of the glycaemic regulation for the development of late-diabetic complications, in which Denmark and the other Scandinavian countries came to occupy a leading place with clinical, randomized studies: the Steno studies, the Oslo study and later the Stockholm study. These were small but showed for the first time that it was possible to attain strict glycaemic regulation over a longer period. In the "Steno 1 study", which was the first prospective, randomized study in the world, multiple injections were compared with insulin pump treatment in 32 patients with simplex retinopathy (incipient diabetic eye disease) [1]. Insulin was mixed individually for each patient, since the pump (Mill-Hill 1001 HM) could infuse at only one speed. The inception of the treatment took place during 7 days' admission to Steno Memorial Hospital. Basal insulin comprised 55 % of the daily insulin dose. HbA_{1c} in the two groups was 68 and 86 % in the first year. The first results were published in 1981 in the Lancet [1].

A reduction in the development of albuminura was found, but no effect on retinopathy, and in fact the data almost showed a deterioration. The occurrence of hypoglycaemia and ketoacidosis was not found to be different in the two groups. All patients in the pump group had technical problems with the pump, and 14 patients had the pump rebuilt from one to five times. Furthermore, there were both technical difficulties with the butterfly in the subcutis and occasional local infections. The pump treatment also illustrated that ketoacidosis developed quickly when the insulin depot in the subcutis was small. In 1986, a new pump study was published from Steno Memorial Hospital, in which 36 patients with microalbuminuria were randomized for treatment with conventional insulin treatment or pump [2, 3]. Five patients in the conventionally treated group developed diabetic kidney disease

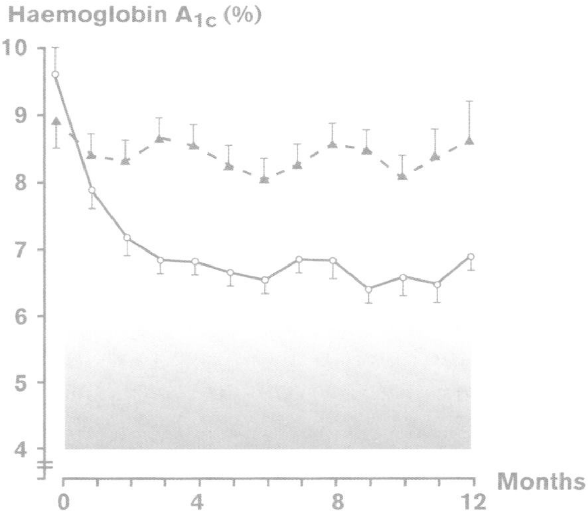

Haemoglobin A_{1c} (%)
10
9
8
7
6
5
4
0
4
8
12
Months

The Steno Study 1981: HbA_{1c} before and during a two year trial in patients with type 1 diabetes with and without insulin pump. (Danish Medical Bulletin, 1985).

against none in the pump group. HbA_{1c} in the two groups was 7.2 and 8.6 %. No difference in retinopathy between the two groups was found, but a tendency for deterioration after 1 year in the pump group was observed. A new concept was introduced, "the point of no return", after which it was not possible to stop the development of the late-diabetic complications.

In 1985, the "Oslo study" showed that quick normalization of the concentration of blood glucose could lead to a transient deterioration in the retinopathy after 3-6 months [4]. A 41-month follow-up on the Oslo study was unable to show that good regulation reduced the progression of retinopathy, but as in the Steno study, the progression in albuminura (egg white in the urine) was reduced in the pump group [5]. Both the Oslo and Steno studies were characterized by insufficient statistical strength and too few patients. In 1984, Århus published a study that described the effect of pump treatment on the intermediary metabolism. Life quality was improved during insulin pump treatment. It was also shown here that strict glycaemic regulation reduced the microalbuminuria [6]. The Kroc study from the USA also found a progression in diabetic eye disease after 8 months' pump treatment.

The fact that it was now technically possible to normalize the blood glucose concentration meant that one could investigate the effect of good metabolic regulation on the beta-cell function, which, as shown in a major Danish study, was preserved to a certain extent in many patients with type 1 diabetes [7]. Insulin pump treatment (strict glycaemic regulation) compared with conventional treatment did not improve the residual (remaining) beta-cell function measured 30 months after diagnosis. On the other hand, full remission (honeymoon) was achieved in the course of 1-2 weeks after diagnosis [7]. This and subsequent studies were the first studies on humans that showed that the concept "glucotoxicity" existed.

These studies were made possible by the development of a sensitive and specific immunoassay for the measurement of C-peptide. The analysis was developed by Lise G Heding at Novo and evaluated in detail by Ole Faber and Christian Binder. The analysis was unique to measure the type 1 patient's own production of insulin during insulin treatment [7]. A large number of studies described the natural history of the residual beta-cell function in type 1 diabetes and what factors were important for the preservation of the function. One of the most surprising finds was that even after many years of diabetes, 10-20 % of the patients had a residual beta-cell function that protected against the development of ketoacidosis and was of importance for the glucagon response to hypoglycaemia, the insulin dose and the degree of glycaemic regulation [7].

Furthermore, a standardized test was developed for measuring the beta-cell function – the glucagon test – which was quick, without adverse effects, and which led to a result that was comparable to a physiological meal test [8]. It is still in use in order to evaluate whether a patient has type 1 or type 2 diabetes [7, 8].

Hypoglycaemia as a barrier to good regulation

Hypoglycaemia is a feared complication among insulin-treated patients, and often the limiting factor to obtaining good glycaemic regulation, also in patients treated with the insulin pump. At the end of the 1970s, a number of studies were carried out at Hvidøre Hospital, in which the functional interaction between the different types of cells in the islets of Langerhans was described in different groups of type 1 patients. It was shown that a residual beta-cell function meant that the glucagon response was preserved during hypoglycaemia [7], and moreover that the response of pancreatic polypeptide during hypoglycaemia could be used as a marker for whether the patients had an autonomous neuropathy (disease in the autonomous nervous system) [9]. Patients with autonomous neuropathy had no glucagon response and a reduced adrenalin response during hypoglycaemia. Later studies showed that the latter group of patients had, on the other hand, an increased sensitivity to adrenalin.

In the 1980s, a number of important clinical studies of type 1 diabetes and hypoglycaemia were carried out at Steno Memorial Hospital. Only approx. 15 % of the type 1 patients had symptoms with a blood glucose < 3.0 mmol/l, and 1/3 of the patients had symptoms of hypoglycaemia without having low blood glucose [10]. The concepts of symptomatic and biochemical hypoglycaemia were introduced. It was

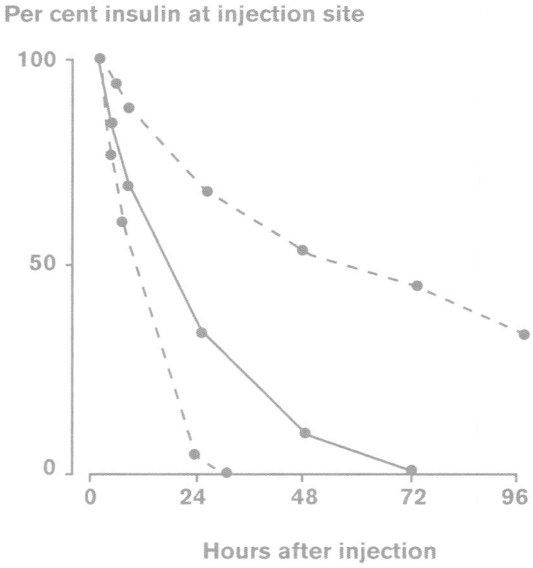

Range of insulin absorption in % of injected NPH insulin in the same patient from day to day. (Diabetologia, 1979).

also shown that the symptoms of hypoglycaemia vary among patients and with the duration of the diabetes. Approx. 40 % of the patients did not have warning symptoms after 30 years' diabetes. The expression "hypoglycaemic unawareness" was, however, introduced only later. Other studies at Steno Memorial Hospital surprisingly showed that approx. 30 % of the patients had nocturnal hypoglycaemia without symptoms and without memory of the episode [11]. The studies led to rules of thumb for how high blood glucose should be before bedtime if hypoglycaemia was to be avoided. Low blood glucose in the morning was also compatible with a high risk of nocturnal hypoglycaemia [11]. The latter was interpreted as a refutation of the "Somogyi effect". This was a misunderstanding. Somogyi has never put forward the view that nocturnal hypoglycaemia leads to increased morning blood glucose, but rather that treatment of the patient with too high insulin doses can lead to labile diabetes with intermittent hypoglycaemia, and that the correct treatment is a reduction of the insulin dose.

The importance of DCCT and EDIC for intensified insulin treatment

The aforementioned pioneering studies of good glycaemic regulation and the risk of developing late-diabetic complications have largely been forgotten today, which shows the risk of conducting small and short studies. It was, however, these studies that inspired and provided arguments for carrying out a sufficiently large study of whether primary intervention could prevent the development of complications.

This study – DCCT (Diabetes Control and Complications Trial) – was published in 1993 [12]. In DCCT, 1,441 patients were randomized for strict glycaemic regulation or for conventional treatment. On average, the patients were followed for 6.5 years and the average HbA_{1c} was 7.3 % in the intensively treated group and 9.2 % in the conventionally treated group. The occurrence of the late-diabetic complications, with both primary and secondary intervention, was halved in the group with strict glycaemic regulation. The study also showed that strict glycaemic regulation was closely and conversely associated with an increased risk of hypoglycaemia.

EDIC (Epidemiology of Diabetes Interventions and Complications), which is the follow-up on DCCT for up to 10 years, has given valuable information on what has been called "metabolic programming" [13]. In the follow-up period, the two groups in DCCT had the same HbA_{1c} (approx. 8.0–8.2 %), while the progression of the late-diabetic complications was largely unchanged from that observed in DCCT and closely associated with HbA_{1c} during DCCT [13]. EDIC shows the importance of being in good glycaemic regulation from the time of diagnosis. Subsequently, the group around Sutherland from Minneapolis published that at 10 years after a pancreas transplantation with normoglycaemia, the diabetic kidney changes had decreased significantly. The discussion whether glycaemic regulation had an effect on the development of the late-diabetic complications was over. The focus now changed to how good regulation could be achieved without too great a risk of hypoglycaemia.

The situation for insulin pump treatment in 2007

In Denmark, today, approx. 550 adults and approx. 220 children, corresponding to 12 % of all children with type 1 diabetes, are receiving insulin pump treatment. The treatment is expensive and time-consuming. In Denmark, a pump costs from DKK 25,000 to DKK 37,000 to purchase and up to DKK 24,000 per year for infusion pipes, monitoring apparatus, etc. What is gained in terms of saved costs for treatment of the late-diabetic complications is not at present known.

There is probably more than one reason why so few patients are in insulin pump treatment in Denmark: bad experiences from the earlier pump era in the form of severe hypoglycaemias and ketoacidoses. Furthermore, it is still not clear who is to pay for the insulin pump treatment. Today, the costs are paid by the departments in which the patients are followed. The pumps are today more reliable in operation, and the most advanced pumps can infuse insulin and at the same time measure the concentration of blood glucose on-line, and they have inbuilt alarms that are activated by too low or too high blood glucose concentrations. In the coming years, a marked increase in the number of pump-treated patients must be expected.

Insulin analogues and intensified treatment of type 1 diabetes

Some departments switched all their patients to treatment with the quick-acting insulin analogues, when these were introduced. Others thought that the analogues did not improve the glycaemic regulation, were more expensive and might induce cell division or cell transformation (mitogenesis). Studies from the first many years after the introduction of the quick-acting analogues showed fewer hypoglycaemia episodes, but no improvement in HbA_{1c}. The problem was perhaps that the new analogues were used like conventional insulin, i.e. as a quick-acting analogue before each main meal and NPH insulin at the evening meal or at bedtime. Today, when the quick-acting analogues, especially *Levemir®*, are combined with basal insulin twice daily, we see not only fewer hypoglycaemia episodes, but also a fall in HbA_{1c}. This is due to a better basal insulin concentration between meals along with a smaller day-to-day variation in the effect of the analogue on hyperglycaemia. The last-mentioned observation has led to the majority of type 1 diabetes patients being treated today with one or more insulin analogues. An advantage of the quick-acting insulin analogues is that they are administered just before the beginning of a meal, while the quick-acting human insulin preparations are best taken 20–30 minutes before a meal. Snacks between meals can often be omitted when using analogue insulin. It has not been clarified whether the 1–2 mmol/l with which quick-acting analogue insulin further reduces the postprandial rise in glucose has an effect on the development of the late-diabetic complications and of cardiovascular disease. In a few years, there will probably be only a few patients who are treated with the conventional insulin preparations.

Intensified treatment of type 2 diabetes

In the 1970s and 1980s, there was no great interest in type 2 diabetes in Denmark. The view was that this disease belonged in general practice. The focus was too much on lifestyle changes with a view to weight loss and increased exercise, most frequently without success. Especially the treatment of the cardiovascular risk factors was not optimal, because in the 1980s and at the start of the 1990s, both diabetologists and cardiologists were uncertain regarding the use and effect of statins. The breakthrough for the statins came with the publication of the 4S study in 1994, where a post hoc analysis showed that the type 2 diabetes patient had a significant effect from treatment with statins. The antihypertensive treatment fared better as both in Århus and in Copenhagen there was a tradition of treating aggressively on the basis of the experience from type 1 diabetes and kidney disease.

There have been astonishingly few investigator-initiated studies of type 2 diabetes in Denmark. In 2001, a study was published in which newly diagnosed type 2 patients were randomized in general practice for conventional treatment or for a more structured treatment respectively. The project was based on further training of the general practitioners and on clear clinical guidelines [14]. Approx. 650 patients were randomized to each group. After 6 years lower fasting blood glucose, HbA_{1c}, and systolic blood pressure were found in the intensively treated group. The consumption of medicine was the same in both groups, except for metformin, which was more used in the intensive group. No difference was found in the development of late-diabetic complications and cardiovascular disease. One of the problems with the study was that the patients were treated according to the same guidelines in the two groups. Thus, fewer than 5 % of the patients, irrespective of group, were given treatment with a statin preparation.

A Danish study has been of very great importance for the treatment of type 2 diabetes [15]. In the Steno 2 study, 160 patients with type 2 diabetes with microalbuminuria were randomized either to aggressive treatment of all risk factors or to conventional treatment [15]. The patients were followed for 8 years. The intensively treated group achieved better glycaemic regulation and lower LDL and blood pressure than the conventionally treated group. It did not prove possible to achieve smoking cessation in the two groups in spite of a very comprehensive and highly structured effort. Changes of weight were not different in the two groups and both groups increased their weight. After 8 years, the occurrence of diabetic kidney disease, eye disease, autonomous neuropathy and cardiovascular disease decreased by approx. 50 % in the intensively treated group. No effect on peripheral neuropathy was found. The Steno 2 study is still the only study in which aggressive multifactorial treatment has been evaluated. Whether the Steno 2 study can be transferred to general practice has not been clarified. The treatment is expensive and complicated, for example the average intake of pills in combination with insulin in the intensively group was 16–17 per day.

The main problem today is not the lack of clinical guidelines for how the type 2 diabetes patient should be treated but to get them implemented in everyday practice. Thus, a recent Danish study from general practice in 2006 showed that only 25–30 % of the type 2 diabetes patients had an LDL cholesterol under 3.0 mmol/l, and that only 30 % were in treatment with statins. Approx. 20 % had a blood pressure under 130/85 mmHg, and about 30 % had achieved the glycaemic goal with an $HbA_{1c} < 6.5$ %. In 2001, 8 % of the patients in Århus County were in treatment with polypharmacy comprising peroral antidiabetica, antihypertensive preparations and lipid-lowering medicine. Too few patients are thus in aggressive pharmacological treatment, and many patients treated with, for instance, statins, are receiving too small doses.

There is therefore a need for more knowledge as to how a targeted introduction, acceptance and use of clinical guidelines can be optimally realised in general practice. One way of improving the treatment in general practice could be an "indicator project", in which cardiovascular risk factors enter as a variable. HbA_{1c}, ophthalmologist checks, and kidney and foot status should be natural indicators in connection with diabetes mellitus. Such projects have been implemented with success in other countries and have resulted in improved treatment.

Concluding comments

Comparing the treatment today with that given in the period 1960–80, we can see that major advances have taken place so that patients now develop fewer late-diabetic complications and more rarely develop cardiovascular disease. Controlled clinical studies from Denmark were the first to show that good glycaemic regulation is crucial for the prognosis in both type 1 and type 2 diabetes. Good regulation can be achieved in more than one way, at any rate in scientific studies. The impression is, however, that in the last many years, no improvement has taken place in the HbA_{1c} level despite good algorithms for aggressive titration of insulin doses and repeated therapy with insulin analogues. The gain has primarily been a reduction in the risk of hypoglycaemia and, with *Levemir®*, a lower increase in weight. Because of technical developments in insulin pumps, the number of persons in insulin pump treatment will rise. So far in Denmark, this treatment has been for the chosen few type 1 diabetes patients, often patients who were already well regulated and with high medicine compliance with the prescribed treatment. What it will be possible to achieve with the new and better pumps, which can at the same time monitor the blood glucose and warn the patient of too high or too low blood glucose levels via inbuilt alarms, is not yet known. There is much to indicate that the solution for improved glycaemic regulation in type 1 diabetes may be medicotechnical, possibly in the form of a close-loop between insulin delivery and blood glucose measurement built into the pump.

The Steno 2 study has had major international impact on the treatment of type 2 diabetes. The study is still the only one that has pointed to the value of multifactorial treatment of a number of cardiovascular risk factors. The study showed that multifactorial treatment is possible in the regime of a scientific investigation, but whether the concept can be implemented in general practice and in the diabetes outpatient clinic is still a matter of debate. It will probably demand a changed attitude to pharmacological treatment and a better understanding of how the patient's compliance with a treatment that consists of 10-20 tablets distributed over 3-4 times a day can be improved. Lifestyle changes alone will never be sufficient for this group of patients, and pharmacological treatment must be started immediately after diagnosis. It continues to be of interest to test the concept of a polypill that contains a number of antihypertensive preparations, a statin and acetylsalicylic acid in a clinical regime in persons with type 2 diabetes.

There is still a great need for well planned studies to investigate how lifestyle changes can best be implemented and maintained. It is important to recognise that lifestyle intervention is also expensive as it is a lifelong process.

There will be focus on new weight-regulating pharmaceuticals and obesity surgery. Especially the type 2 diabetes patient can benefit from obesity surgery in relation to life quality, morbidity and mortality. Type 2 diabetes may very well become a "major surgical disease". Thus, obesity surgical interventions are today the most rapidly growing among surgical procedures in the USA.

Danish diabetological research has in terms of the number of publications and their impact had a very strong position internationally. As will have appeared from the present chapter, this does not, however, apply to clinical intervention research, in which there have been astonishingly few investigator-initiated studies published from Denmark. This is disappointing as especially our infrastructure and our treatment system could have been expected to promote clinical intervention research. But this can be remedied now when a large proportion of the "Globalisation Funds" are to be used on "patient-oriented" clinical research that will benefit the patient.

REFERENCES

1. *Effect of 6 months of strict metabolic control on eye and kidney function in insulin dependent diabetics with background retinopathy. Steno Study Group. Lancet 1982;i:121-4.*
2. *Feldt-Rasmussen B, Mathiesen ER, Deckert T. Effect of two years of strict metabolic control on progression of incipient nephropathy in insulin-dependent diabetes. Lancet 1986;ii:1300-4.*
3. *Feldt-Rasmussen B, Mathiesen ER, Hegedüs L, Deckert T. Kidney function during 12 months of strict metabolic control in insulin-dependent diabetic patients with incipient nephropathy. N Engl J Med 1986;314:665-70.*
4. *Dahl-Jørgensen K, Brinckmann-Hansen O, Hanssen KF, Norman N. Rapid Tightening of blood glucose control leads to transient deterioration of retinopathy in insulin-dependent diabetes mellitus. Br Med J 1985;290:811-5.*
5. *Dahl-Jørgensen K, Hanssen KF, Kierulf P, Bjoro T, Sandvik L, Aagenaes O. Reduction of albumin excretion after 4 years of continuous subcutaneous insulin infusion in insulin-dependent diabetes mellitus. Acta Endocrinol (Copenh) 1988;117:19-25.*
6. *Beck-Nielsen H, Richelsen B, Mogensen CE, Olsen T, Ehlers N, Nielsen CB, Charles P. Effect of pump treatment for one year on renal function and retinal morphology in patients with IDDM. Diabetes Care 1985;8:585-9.*

7. *Madsbad S. Prevalence of residual B cell function and its metabolic consequences in Type 1 (insulin-dependent) diabetes. Diabetologia 1983;24:141-7.*
8. *Faber OK, Binder C. C-peptide response to glucagon. A test for the residual beta-cell function in diabetes mellitus. Diabetes 1977;26:605-10.*
9. *Krarup T, Schwartz TW, Hilsted J, Madsbad S, Overlaege O, Sestoft L. Impaired response of pancreatic polypeptide to hypoglycaemia: an early sign of autonomic neuropathy in diabetics. Br Med J 1979;2:1544-6.*
10. *Pramming S, Thorsteinsson B, Bendtson I, Binder C. The relationship between symptomatic and biochemical hypoglycaemia in insulin-dependent diabetic patients. J Intern Med 1990;228:641-6.*
11. *Pramming S, Thorsteinsson B, Bendtson I, Ronn B, Binder C. Nocturnal hypoglycaemia in patients receiving conventional treatment with insulin. Br Med J (Clin Res Ed) 1985;10;291:376-9.*
12. *The Diabetes Control and Complications Trial Research Group. The effect of intensive treatment of diabetes on the development and progression of long-term complications in insulin-dependent diabetes mellitus. N Engl J Med 1993;329:977-86.*
13. *The Writing Team for the Diabetes Control and Complications Trial/Epidemiology of Diabetes Interventions and Complications Research group. Effect of intensive therapy on the microvascular complications of type 1 diabetes mellitus. JAMA 2002;287:2563-9.*
14. *Olivarius NF, Beck-Nielsen H, Andreasen AH, Horder M, Pedersen PA. Randomised controlled trial of structured personal care of type 2 diabetes mellitus. BMJ 2001;323:970-5.*
15. *Gæde P, Vedel P, Larsen N, Jensen GV, Parving HH, Pedersen OB. Multifactorial intervention and cardiovascular disease in patients with type 2 diabetes. N Engl J Med 2003;348:383-93.*

THE RELATION BETWEEN BLOOD GLUCOSE AND HbA_{1C} – A DANISH PIONEERING EFFORT

JENS SANDAHL CHRISTIANSEN

Introduction

In the last half of the 1970s, graph paper, rubbers and pencils were in high demand at the clinical departments in Denmark that were interested in analyzing the blood glucose profiles of patients with insulin-dependent diabetes mellitus.

Computers as we know them today were at a very early stage of development, took up many square metres of floor space and were difficult to gain access to. Small portable calculating machines were a help when we had to work out the correlations between X and Y, but a very substantial part of the analysis of the blood glucose profiles consisted of entering the data onto graph paper and calculating mean blood glucose (MBG), mean amplitude of glycaemic excursions (MAGE), Schlichtkrull's M-value, etc. At Steno Memorial Hospital (SMH), various clinical research projects had been initiated with a view to optimizing glycaemic regulation, including the development of prototypes for insulin pumps (initially for intravenous use), and trials with the country's first artificial pancreas gland (*Biostator®*) were in process [1]. There was therefore a need for an evaluation of the patients' glycaemic regulation both in the short and long term. All these measures required a major and painstaking effort based on calculations of the registered blood glucose values.

In 1976, Ronald Koenig and his group published their observation of the correlation between the blood glucose regulation and HbA_{1c} in diabetes patients [2]. This groundbreaking work was soon followed up by Boas Gonen from Chicago, who published corresponding data the following year [3]. Suddenly, we found ourselves with completely different possibilities of documenting the average glycaemic regulation in our patients with the help of a single blood sample – a possibility that meant a revolution in clinical diabetes research, initially for type 1 diabetes but later also for type 2 diabetes.

Background

The demonstration that HbA_{1c} could be used as a reliable marker of the average glycaemic regulation came at a very convenient moment. The discovery of insulin and its first clinical use in 1922, whereby the survival of patients with type 1 diabetes beyond 6 months became possible, was followed by the observation of so-called late-diabetic complications in the form of microangiopathy – disease in small blood vessels – in the retina, kidneys and nerve tissue. From the Danish side, Knud Lundbæk published a paper in The Lancet in the early 1950s demonstrating a link between retinopathy, nephropathy and neuropathy – disorders of the eyes, kidneys and nerves – showing them to be one specific vascular disease.

The relation between the degree of glycaemic regulation and the development of late-diabetic manifestations was not clear. Purely intuitively, many people felt that there had to be a link, while others maintained that patients with type 1 diabetes had a tendency to develop microangiopathy at the same time – a tendency that was independent of the diabetes and of the glycaemic regulation. Thus, in the 1960s, Marvin Siperstein thought he could show that the basal membrane had become thicker in type 1 diabetes patients already by the time of diagnosis, which made it reasonable to assume that the damage would have happened irrespective of the development of hyperglycaemia [4]. Siperstein's observation was, as mentioned elsewhere, later refuted in Denmark by Ruth Østerbye and her group.

However, the clinical reality meant that while attempting a near-normalization of blood glucose in these patients, one induced hypoglycaemia – a clinical complication that is and was feared by patients and medical staff alike. American researchers in particular maintained that there were no reasonable grounds for exposing patients to this risk inasmuch as it had not been proved that the development of late-diabetic complications could be prevented or delayed by the near-normalization of blood glucose [5]. European researchers, however, more and more frequently proposed that there had to be such a link. This was based on the findings of retrospective studies.

Pirart from Belgium did a huge job in registering and monitoring a patient cohort that he followed personally, which led to three reports based on observations from 1947 to 1973 [6]. Here he presented substantial evidence – albeit retrospective – that good metabolic regulation was associated with partial protection against or delay of the development of the late-diabetic syndrome.

In the earlier 1970s, studies of the natural history of type 1 diabetes patients had been started up at Steno Memorial Hospital on the initiative of Jacob Poulsen and Torsten Deckert. These studies led to the conclusion that frequent contact with a centre with diabetological expertise ensured a better prognosis – regarding both the development of complications and of the patient's quality of life [7]. Poulsen and Deckert's observations gave rise to a good deal of muted dissatisfaction round about in the kingdom, since it was felt – justifiably or not – that these prognosis works were the reflection of a certain feeling of self-sufficiency at SMH, and also that they implied an indirect criticism of diabetes care elsewhere.

Seen with contemporary eyes, it must of course be conceded that the cohort studies of that time were scarcely representative and could in no circumstances be taken to indicate to what extent the degree of metabolic regulation had an effect on the development of complications.

Today, however, most people would agree with the chief message from these prognostic studies, namely that the extent of diabetic care offered and received has an effect on the prognosis of type 1 diabetes.

The need for documentation of treatment results

In the mid-1970s, Danish diabetology was buzzing with research activity in the field of late-diabetic complications. Deckert and Poulsen's prognosis studies for type 1 diabetes patients, Jørgen Pedersen's calculation of the results from treatment of pregnant diabetes patients along with national and international analyses of the effect of laser treatment on retinopathy showed with all desirable clarity that it was possible to exert a favourable influence on the course of the disease. In Denmark, the focus was on the possible effects of blood pressure treatment and on the possibilities of improved glycaemic regulation with the help of optimized insulin treatment. In respect of the administration of insulin, a number of parallel measures were taking place under the leadership of Torsten Deckert with attempts at developing intravenous insulin infusion pumps (Lørup and Deckert) and the purchase of the first mass-produced artificial pancreas – the *Biostator®*. Both at SMH and at Hvidøre, intensive studies were in progress to further illuminate insulin absorption (injected subcutaneously) (Binder and later Køhlendorf, Lauritzen and Hildebrandt).

In the daily press, the arrival of the *Biostator®* gave rise to much attention. For example, Bent Henius – a journalist and diabetes patient of many years – chose to do a feature on TV. I clearly remember that prior to the recordings for this news item I had a very direct talk with Henius with what I myself considered to be the very sensible aim of ensuring that the news of this artificial pancreas was not proclaimed as the final, immediately accessible solution for all type 1 diabetes patients. Henius stuck fully to the agreed conditions, but clearly felt my behaviour to be somewhat patronising – in view of my youth. He had his small revenge by consistently referring to me in the item – both in writing and orally – as professor,

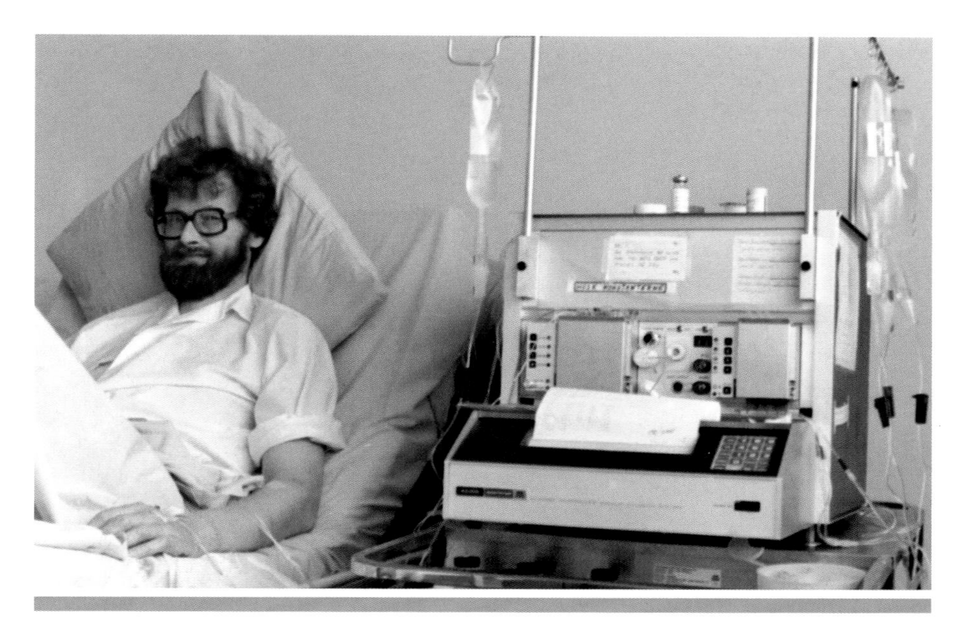

Patient connected to a Biostator®, *which besides being able to measure blood glucose could be programmed to administer insulin and glucose. The patient is* not *Bent Henius (see text).*

consultant, DMSc, which naturally gave rise to a good deal of amusement at my expense at SMH.

At a subsequent Open House arrangement at SMH, the hospital was almost swamped by more than 3000 people who wanted to see the artificial pancreas. Henius had made himself available for the arrangement, and the many visitors could meet the journalist placed in a hospital bed linked to the *Biostator®*, talking uninterruptedly and enthusiastically about the new era in diabetes treatment. There was not much substance in the latter claim, but at least the hospital had acquired a valuable instrument that we could use for a more precise evaluation of the glycaemic regulation.

In 1978, Pickup and Keen from Guy's Hospital in London proposed the use of continuous subcutaneous infusion of insulin with the help of small portable pumps as a feasible way forward. It soon became clear that when using this principle, it would probably be possible to achieve a clear improvement of the average glycaemic regulation – and hereby to investigate whether this would have a crucial influence on the development of late complications. At Steno Memorial Hospital, the possibility was briefly considered of entering into an English-American multi-centre study sponsored by the Kroc Foundation. However, Deckert decided that the hospital itself had the requisite funds and possibilities, and the Steno 1 Pump Study – the first prospective study that later showed a positive effect from optimized glycaemic regulation – was launched.

But how should the treatment relating to the effect on the mean blood glucose concentration be documented?

At this time, outpatients at SMH had blood glucose measured postprandially (after a meal) in the morning and glucose secretion in a specimen of 24-hour urine as the main cornerstones of their treatment. But this did not contain much documentation of what happened during the rest of the 24 hours. However, at this time, there had now appeared reasonably simple and patient-friendly devices that made home monitoring of blood glucose possible, although the precision of these measurements still left something to be desired. The measurement of glucose in 24-hour urine continued to be regarded as a reasonably good method for documenting how often during the 24 hours the blood glucose had been above the kidney threshold. The day-to-day variation in the glucose secretion was, however, enormous, and it was of course not practical to imagine that a patient would have to be constantly collecting urine in order to document the glycaemic regulation over a longer period.

HbA_{1c} – the great leap forward

Understandably, the description of a possible link between HbA_{1c} and the mean blood glucose concentration evoked enormous attention – also in Denmark. At Steno Memorial Hospital, laboratory chief Per Aaby Svendsen promptly began to try to document the validity of this new parameter, which was after all almost too

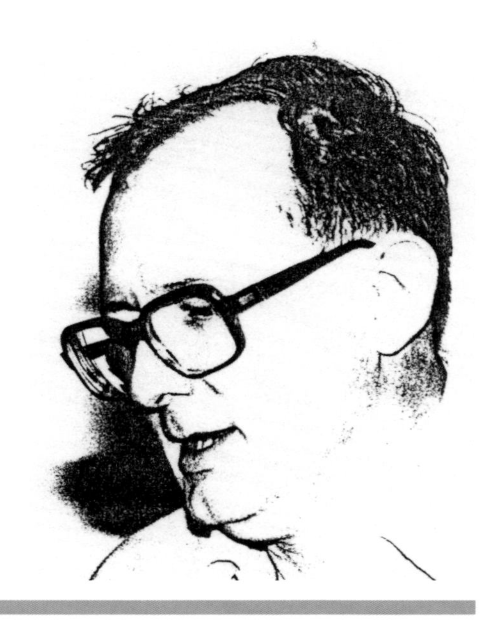

Per Aaby Svendsen (1982) was an international pioneer in the investigation of HbA_{1c} and in the clinical use of its measurement in blood.

good to be true. Aaby ran the clinical routine laboratory work with great effectiveness at the hospital. His attention to detail, sense of order and focus on quality assurance (before this word had yet been invented in its political sense) were legendary. He had grown up on Bornholm, which could be clearly heard when he raised his voice – something that despite his pronounced temperament he did only after having considered things thoroughly. He was a very modest and private person, who nonetheless exhibited an immediate openness and obligingness to new staff. Many a hopeful young researcher would later think back with gratitude on how he patiently introduced them to basic laboratory techniques (and conduct).

Per Aaby Svendsen threw himself with great energy and expertise into the testing and development of methods. Thus, he was the first to show that it was possible both *in vivo* and *in vitro* to change the concentration of glycated haemoglobin within a few hours [8]. This observation explained why HbA_{1c} had been found to vary considerably when one had – accidentally – carried out a measurement with a few weeks', indeed even days' interval. Aaby solved the problem by preincubation of the samples and thereby avoided interference from the "rapid" part of HbA_{1c}. The measurements thus became more precise than before this knowledge was available, and this work created the foundation for the important American-headed work that led to the standardisation programme that has made possible comparisons between laboratory measurements all over the world and thereby reporting in articles of comparable HbA_{1c} values. Aaby and his co-workers at the clinic also tackled the comprehensive, time-demanding job of trying to determine a more exact link between HbA_{1c} and the real mean glucose value

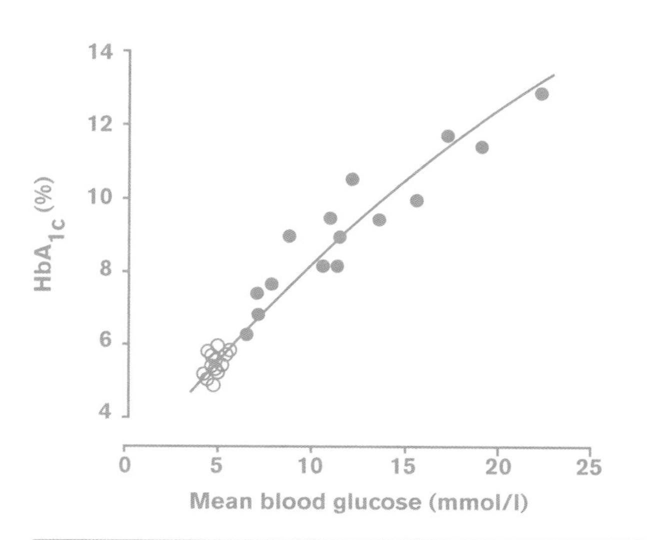

Per Aaby Svendsen's results concerning the link between the mean blood glucose concentration and HbA_{1c}. The graph is calculated using the regression equation $HbA_{1c} = 2.07 \times \text{mean blood glucose}^{0.596}$.

over time. In connection with the planning of the Steno 1 Pump Study, it was decided that – at any rate in the introductory period – the patients should document their blood glucose values with the help of frequent samples taken with small capillary tubes at home, which were then sent by ordinary post to SMH.

The capillary tube method was used for the collection of thousands of blood glucose values, and Aaby and his colleagues hereby succeeded in describing the link between HbA_{1c} and mean blood glucose. The HbA_{1c} value could thus be "translated" into an average blood glucose value that the patients could relate to [9]. The method for determining HbA_{1c} was slow, and in time as both clinical and research needs demanded more and more measurements, Aaby had to make use of his inventiveness and well-known technical ingenuity. People who worked there remember how the fume cupboard was for a period filled up with long rows of Trivelli columns, which made it possible for Aaby to increase the analysis capacity considerably. In that process, Aaby received invaluable help from laboratory technicians Birthe Lørup and Ulla Søegaard. Systematic work on the clinical use of HbA_{1c} was also taking place elsewhere in Denmark. Thus, in Glostrup researchers were engaged in a comprehensive and systematic project in the paediatric segment (Henrik B Mortensen), while data were published from Århus and Odense that documented the usefulness of HbA_{1c} in patient education.

The publication of two large prospective foreign studies – DCCT [10] and UKPDS [11] – of type 1 and type 2 diabetes patients respectively demonstrating the beneficial effect of good average glucose regulation on the development of late-diabetic complications put an end to the many years of discussion of this question. Since then, HbA_{1c} and changes in it have been a primary parameter in all kinds of intervention study in which change of the glycaemic regulation has been attempted, just as HbA_{1c} is also a natural and necessary part of the description of any kind of patient material in a clinical study – irrespective of the aim of the study. Today, the health authorities have accepted HbA_{1c} and changes in it as a surrogate variable for the development of late-diabetic complications. Nevertheless, over the years, there have been persistent problems with the standardization of the method of measurement, which has varied from country to country and from laboratory to laboratory. Relatively recently, it has proved possible to develop a method for the determination of "genuine HbA_{1c}" (the glycocylization degree of the N-terminal amino acid valin in the haemoglobin molecule's beta-chain). In this way, a "gold standard" for HbA_{1c} measurement has been identified. All commercial methods for HbA_{1c} determination calibrate to it, and an actual international standardization has thereby been implemented. In addition, the final determination of the link between HbA_{1c}

and the mean blood glucose concentration over a long period of time is now possible.

This project is now well underway in a cooperation among groups in Europe and the USA under the leadership of a steering group set up jointly by EASD, ADA and IDF. The results have been presented at the 43rd Meeting of EASD in Amsterdam 2007. The initiative for this was Danish and started in Jørn Nerup's period as EASD president. This work leads directly back to the pioneering work in which Per Aaby Svendsen was the driving force more than 20 years ago.

Limitations and possibilities

As already described, the introduction of HbA_{1c} measurement has had a colossal importance for both clinical and research work in the field of type 1 and type 2 diabetes.

The fact that some patients unfortunately experience a quicker development of complications in their disease despite good HbA_{1c} values, just as the opposite is fortunately also the case, has stimulated a discussion of the limited clinical value of the HbA_{1c} measurements. Thus, it is today a fairly widespread view that not only the average blood glucose value over 24 hours, expressed as HbA_{1c}, but also the extent and frequency of the glycaemic fluctuations are of importance for the development of late-diabetic complications. The development of macroangiopathy in patients with type 2 diabetes is thus asserted by many to be closely associated with the degree of glycaemic fluctuations – e.g. postprandially. There are also advocates of the view that by comparing good measurements for the patients' mean blood glucose and the resulting HbA_{1c} concentration in the individual patient, it will be possible to say something about the patient's tendency to glycate proteins and thereby perhaps identify those patients with a particularly high risk of developing micro- and macroangiopathy.

Anyhow, it is becoming increasingly clearer that in the slightly longer term, the measurement of HbA_{1c} is unlikely to stand alone as a parameter in our endeavours to improve the glycaemic regulation and document the effect of treatment. In coming years, the rapid development of methods for more or less continuous glucose registration – invasive or non-invasive – will undoubtedly bring us an increased understanding of the physiology behind the formation of HbA_{1c} and thereby also of this parameter's clinical advantages and limitations.

REFERENCES

1. *Christiansen JS, Svendsen PA, Deckert T. Insulin treatment and state of control before, during and after connection to a glucose controlled insulin infusion system (BIOSTATOR). Horm Metab Res 1979; suppl 8:131-4*
2. *Koenig RJ, Peterson CM, Jones RL, Saudek C, Lehrman M, Cerami A. Correlation of glucose regulation and haemoglobin A1c in diabetes mellitus. N Engl J Med 1976;295:417-20*
3. *Gonen B, Rubenstein AH, Rochman H, Tanega SP, Horwitz DL. Hæmoglobin A1c: An indicator for the metabolic control of diabetic patients. Lancet 1977;ii:734-7*
4. *Siperstein MD, Unger RH, Madison LL. Studies of muscle capillary basement membranes in normal subjects, diabetic and prediabetic patients. J Clin Invest 1968;47:1973-99*
5. *Siperstein MD, Foster DW, Knowles HC Jr., Levine R, Madison LL, Roth J. Control of blood glucose and diabetic vascular disease. N Engl J Med 1977;296:1060-3*
6. *Pirart J. Diabetes mellitus and its degenerative complications: a prospective study of 4.400 patients observed between 1947 and 1973 (in three parts). Diabete Metab 1977;3:97-107; 173-82; 245-56*
7. *Deckert T, Poulsen JE. Prognosis for juvenile diabetics with late diabetic manifestations. Diabetologia 1978;14: 363-370*
8. *Svendsen PA, Christiansen JS, Søegaard U, Welinder BS, Nerup J. Rapid changes in chromatographically determined haemoglobin A1c induced by short-term changes in glucose concentration. Diabetologia 1980;19:130-6*
9. *Svendsen PA, Lauritzen T, Søegaard U, Nerup J. Glycosylated haemoglobin and steady-state mean blood glucose concentrations in type 1 (insulin-dependent) diabetes. Diabetologia 1982;23:403-5*
10. *The DCCT Research Group. The effect of intensive treatment of diabetes on the development and progression of long-term complications in insulin-dependent diabetes mellitus. N Engl Med J 1993;329:977-86*
11. *UK Prospective Diabetes Study (UKPDS) Group. Intensive blood-glucose control with sulphonylureas or insulin compared with conventional treatment and risk of complications in patients with type 2 diabetes (UKPDS33). Lancet 1998;352:837-53*

FROM PATERNALISM TO SELF-CARE

TORSTEN LAURITZEN & HELLE TERKILDSEN

Introduction

The title suggests a simple development in the relationship between doctor and patient over time. But, in fact, it has not been that simple. Since the possibility of diet treatment became known and the discovery of insulin, self-care has been a necessary part of diabetes treatment, and, as we shall argue below, paternalism continues to be part of diabetes treatment. The balance between paternalism and self-care has changed concurrently and is probably linked with an extension of the doctor-patient relationship. Today, this is a matter of a relation between the patient and a professional health team consisting of doctors, nurses, dieticians, podiatrists and others.

Historical background

The Nei Ching, probably the oldest medical textbook in the world, is Chinese and from 2600 BC. In the book, it is written that the Chinese doctor wanted to know about how the patient had fallen ill, that is about how the person had offended against Tao (Way of Heaven). To understand this, he took into account the patient's rank, household, economic situation, feeling of wellbeing, appetite, dreams and the weather. In other words, a holistic medicine based on the idea that the patient's care for himself or herself was of importance. Self-care is thus not a new concept.

In Ancient Greece, holistic and patient-centred medicine also enjoyed favourable conditions. When one was to make a diagnosis in Hippocrates' time, one had to form an impression of the patient's lifestyle, housing, work and eating habits. Because of the absence of a possible treatment, the most important part of the physician's work was to make diagnoses and tell the patient what the prognosis was. At the same time, he would – no doubt paternalistically – urge his patients to live sensibly and thereby be responsible for their own self-care.

Definitions:

Paternalism is defined in the Stanford Encyclopedia of Philosophy: *"Paternalism is the interference of a state or an individual with another person, against their will, and justified by a claim that the person interfered with will be better off or protected from harm. The issue of paternalism arises with respect to restrictions by the law such as anti-drug legislation, the compulsory wearing of seatbelts, and in medical contexts by the withholding of relevant information concerning a patient's condition by physicians. At the theoretical level it raises questions of how persons should be treated when they are less than fully rational".*

Central in the above definition are the words 'against their will'. In our opinion *'against their will'* should be understood more broadly, i.e., to include the situation in which the patient feels under strong pressure to do what the health professional wishes.

Self care has appeared in the international literature since 1955 and in Danish literature since 1977. There is no single unambiguous definition, but most definitions stress that the individual must assume responsibility for his or her disease and its treatment. Nurse D Orem, who is the most cited researcher in self care, emphasizes the importance of the support in relation to self care given by health professionals to patients who do not have the necessary resources themselves. In the Danish government's public health programme from 2001, "Healthy Throughout Life" the individual's self care is highlighted as an important factor in prevention, while the health and social services are expected to set the framework that will make it possible for the individual to live healthily with his or her disease. In a recent English textbook on diabetes, self care is specifically defined as appropriate behaviour in respect of diet, physical activity, medicine consumption and daily monitoring.

The holistic approach to illness and treatment was widespread in Denmark right up to the 1920s. The Danish tradition was based on ancient medicine. This is the thinking on which the whole sanatorium movement for the treatment of, for instance, tuberculosis was based. Without an effective medical treatment, the tuberculosis patients took a comprehensive hygienic cure that involved their whole way of life – diet, exercise, topics of conversation, interests, soil conditions, etc. The holistic approach was also applied in explaining the disease – family, interests, clothing, climate, temperament and inheritance were used to explain tuberculosis, even long after the tuberculosis bacteria had been discovered.

Strict diet was the first effective treatment of diabetes – a treatment that required both self-care and self-discipline. Now that diabetes had an effective treatment, paternalism was backed up by authority. The paternalist physician thus came into his own at the end of the 19th century, when, for example, the German diabetes expert Bernhard Naunyn invested much effort and authority in helping his patients to keep to the right diet. Disobedient patients were quite simply locked in their rooms, often for months.

The next decisive step in the treatment of diabetes was the discovery of insulin in 1921. Now the patients' self-care was expanded from strict diet to also including self-injection, boiling needles and treatment of the insulin episodes that were one of the side-effects of insulin.

The Danish consultant, Ebbe Kjems, DMSc, was born in 1920 and relates in his memoirs that as a six-year-old, he got so tired that he could not stand up but had to lie on the floor whenever he got a chance to do so. The family doctor found sugar in his urine, and Ebbe had to live on cabbage morning, noon and night until it was decided that he should consult Dr. H.C. Hagedorn, who together with August Krogh, was the father of the first Danish insulin. Evidently, Hagedorn paternalistically urged self-care on his patient, for Ebbe Kjems continues: "*My father bought me a second-hand bike. (...) On this bike I could*

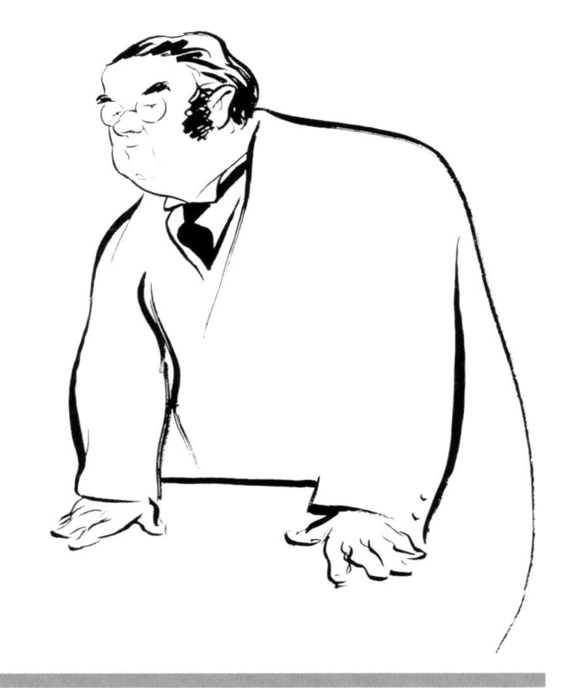

HC Hagedorn – fear- and respect-inspiring – not just for a small boy with diabetes, but also at the defence of a doctoral dissertation.

cycle every fortnight to my check-up with Dr. Hagedorn, who lived on Onsgårdsvej in Hellerup, where he had his surgery. In his rooms, there were test tubes and measuring cylinders. (...) I thought Hagedorn was a giant, and my respect for him was unbounded. Once he said to me: "And now you don't touch the sugar bowl", so when my mother had asked me to lay the table, I washed my hands after carrying the sugar bowl to the table. I decided early that I wanted to be a doctor. (...) My diabetes didn't give me much bother, but it was hard for me to get from school to home and back again in order to eat a head of cabbage between 10.45 and 11.15, and there was a troublesome problem that occurred in connection with a Danish lesson just before the lunch break. Here we did spelling. Words had to be chanted in syllables endlessly repeated, and the monotony in connection with low blood sugar often gave me an unbearable headache."

Dr. Hagedorn, who treated Ebbe Kjems, is quoted for the following statement to another patient: *"You don't need to ask why, when I tell you how!"* Probably an approach that was accepted, but one that could scarcely have strengthened the patient's motivation to take responsibility for his own illness.

In 1932, the first diabetes hospital proper in Denmark, Steno Memorial Hospital, opened. Six years later, it was followed by Hvidøre Hospital, in the beginning as a diabetes sanatorium. The two hospitals were later merged under the name of Steno Diabetes Center. The treatment of patients at these hospitals has undergone a development from paternalism to self-care. This is, for example, reflected in the hospitals' bed capacity, which has been reduced from about 60 to about 10 today. At the same time, there has been a considerable expansion of outpatient activities and an ongoing development of the teaching given to patients on how they can take care of their own treatment by modifying their diets, exercising, monitoring blood sugar, changing their insulin dose and taking medicine for, for example, high blood pressure and cholesterol.

Self-care makes progress

The intentions regarding self-care were clear already in 1938, when Hvidøre Hospital was opened. Thorvald Pedersen, one of Novo's founders, made a speech in which he said: *"In recognition of the fact that the final goal of our work must be to look after the needs of those with diabetes, we have in acquiring Hvidøre wished to make an attempt (...) at creating the best possible conditions for the patients in which they learn to adapt their way of life to the disease. It is incredibly important that they get as detailed knowledge as possible of the special nature and treatment of diabetes."* Afterwards, Hvidøre's chief consultant Harald Hansborg said: *"Diabetes patients who are themselves interested in their treatment will virtually be able to live and do their jobs like any other person. At Hvidøre, we must teach them to understand and participate in the treatment of their disease."*

In 1938, then, it was the goal to teach patients as much about diabetes and its treatment as possible, just as it was a goal that patients should live as normally as possible and themselves take part in the treatment. Here the first seeds for a more explicit discourse on self-care were sown, even though the concept had not been defined, and there was much knowledge that was not yet accessible to health-educational practice.

In the 1970s, this theme was taken up by nurses. By establishing posts for nurses whose only task was to inform, motivate, instruct and help patients to implement diabetes regulation and treatment in their everyday lives, diabetologists in Denmark trod a new path that inspired similar measures for other patient groups with chronic diseases.

There is probably no single factor that has determined the development towards self-care. We shall in the following describe a number of biomedical, technological, health educational, political and societal factors that have in different ways led to this development.

The nature of the disease and the possibilities of treatment

The biomedical development has given greater knowledge of the nature of the disease and the possibilities of treatment and has resulted in the development of numerous medical preparations. Genetic, cellular, psychological and behavioural mechanisms can lead to diabetes. For many years there has, for instance, been focus on the link between obesity and the development of type 2 diabetes. Furthermore, lifestyle habits and a low level of physical activity are connected with diabetes. Intervention in relation to lifestyle and medicine-taking involve self-care.

Technology

In the field of technology, it is especially the new insulins, insulin pens, insulin pumps and devices for self-monitoring of blood sugar that have contributed to the development from paternalism to self-care. Before the 1970s, patients with strongly fluctuating blood sugar had to be admitted so that one could frequently measure their blood sugar throughout the day and night and regulate their insulin. The doctors held conferences with the nurses, who then passed on the insulin changes to the patients. At a conference, it might be mentioned that a patient was often seen at the local grocer's apparently buying confectionary. The view at the conference would be that this was the explanation for the blood sugar fluctuations. But at the same time, the patient was taking part in a scientific study that later showed that insulin absorption from the injection site in the skin was so varied that this explained 80 % of the blood sugar variations. Or, to put it in another way: 80 % of the fluctuations were beyond the patient's control! Seen from a present-day perspective what was at work here was a paternalistic and unnecessary impugnment of the patient that was perhaps both an expression of powerlessness in the face of the inexplicably fluctuating blood sugar levels and also of a frustration at the absence of medical possibilities as well as of a lack of knowledge concerning the instability of insulin absorption! New, faster acting insulin preparations and insulin pumps together with the patients' possibility of monitoring their blood sugar in their daily lives have meant a necessary development towards increased self-care.

From moralising to autonomy in patient treatment

In the 20th century, health education moved from being moralizing/authoritarian towards an approach based on equal partnership. The moralizing aspect has been and is still, in our view, prevalent in parts of the medical

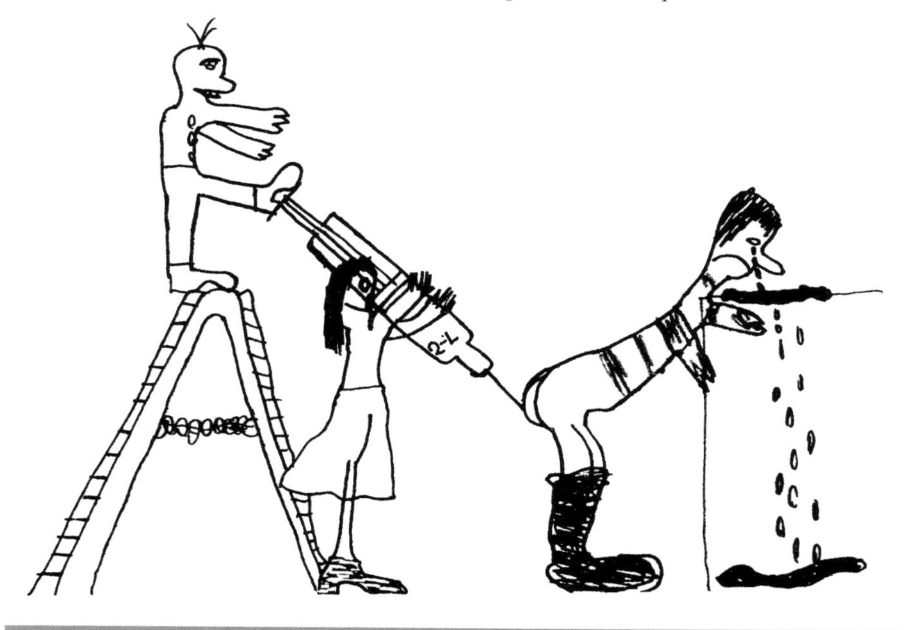

Autonomy and self care is one thing – but a child's view of diabetes and diabetes treatment is often something quite different.
(The child's drawing kindly lent by Vibeke Nerup).

world. Good diabetes regulation signals that the patient is behaving well and has appropriate habits. The treatment is successful, and the self-care satisfactory. On the other hand, poor regulation is ascribed to the fact that the patient's way of living with diabetes has partly failed, and that the self-care is not good enough.

Life with diabetes has been a complex challenge ever since Ebbe Kjems' day. He had to eat his cabbage and was, with his family, the person who had to deal with the consequences and challenges of the disease on a daily basis. Once a fortnight, he received medical assistance from Dr. Hagedorn. Today, both our knowledge about and the prognosis of diabetes have improved, but on the other hand the choices of treatment are now numerous and complex. People with type 1 diabetes must themselves take the responsibility for insulin injections several times a day, for insulin monitoring and for regulating their consumption of food and physical activity in relation to these factors. For a person with type 2 diabetes, the medical treatment may be less challenging, but here great demands are made on the person's diet, exercise and lifestyle in general. The paternalistic and strict diet demands have today been replaced by lifestyle guidelines and principles. At the same time, the prognosis is to a high degree dependent on the patients following the recommended on-going check-ups of, for instance, the eyes, feet, lipids and blood pressure, so that the right preventive measures can be taken.

The Health Service's demands

In present-day Denmark, the Health Service requires the patient to be active and involved. Patients must take responsibility for their own treatment. Health personnel have therefore had to redefine their role and help patients to clarify their own strong sides and resources, so that on the basis of their own set of values, they can take decisions about the treatment. A very important tool for health personnel is communication, for instance "the motivating interview". Ebbe Kjems and his family probably had the strength and resources to take responsibility. His stubbornness in continuing to chant spelling words despite too low blood sugar shows great strength. But we doubt whether everyone with diabetes has the strength to make the required choices. It must be a tremendous challenge for a six-year-old to stick to a healthy diet today when not only the shops, but also our homes, schools and sports halls are filled with fatty and sugary foods.

Self-care and the patient's responsibility are also important elements of the treatment in, for example, the USA, Canada and England. One speaks of being an "expert patient". Just as in Denmark, to be an expert patient means that the individual has control over his or her life and can look after his or her own situation and treatment in collaboration with the health professionals. As an expert patient, one undergoes a patient education in which one acquires the relevant skills.

In 2006, the National Board of Health in Denmark urged all municipalities and regions to offer patient education programmes along the lines of a model from Stanford University: *The Chronic Disease Self-Management Program*, which is based on experience exchange among persons with chronic diseases such as diabetes. The programme realises the idea of self-care, which can probably help some persons with diabetes, but, as we see it, by no means everyone. Some people do not want to sit on the school bench to learn to be an expert patient, and others do not have the necessary mental or social extra resources to participate in such activities. Yet others do not wish to reveal to strangers their victories or defeats in the struggle against obesity. *The Chronic Disease Self-Management Program* is probably a good and inexpensive offer for the Health Service to make, but it does not embrace everyone.

Is self-care modern paternalism?

Slightly critically, one may ask whether the expert patient and self-care are merely in reality a modern form of paternalism, because the Health Service assumes the right to define how the collaboration between health personnel and patient should take place. Is there any possibility at all that the resource-weak patient can take on the responsibility that the Health Service demands? Does the concept mean in its furthest consequence that the health professionals will come into the picture only when the patient's resources have been exhausted? One must hope not!

Perhaps, after all, we have ascribed too much importance to self-care with the risk that poor regulation is regarded as the patient's own fault – "blaming the victim". Self-care alone is not enough! The absorption of sugar from the intestine after eating, the absorption of insulin from the injection site and the hormone-linked increase in blood sugar in the early morning hours (the dawn phenomenon) are some of the physiological factors that cannot be regulated by lifestyle and mentality, and which can result in blood sugar fluctuations that the individual is not in control of. This is knowledge we have had for decades, but which has not been included on an equal footing with self-care as explanations for unsatisfactory blood sugar regulation.

We permit ourselves to doubt whether self-care alone is what the patients want. Perhaps it is also – in disguise – the best that health professionals can come up with to distance themselves from the authoritarian administration of the concept of paternalism, which seems out of step with the general development of society, and which very few people are comfortable with today.

Perhaps self-care is not the right option for old Mrs Jensen, who can easily get the feeling that she is not doing it "well enough". How can she choose between all the many and often conflicting items of information that she receives from those who treat her and from the media. Perhaps she would be more content if she was told what the health professionals think she should do. It is not only the elderly who may find it difficult to understand and deal with the offer of self-care in their treatment. Children and groups with other cultural values, and other perceptions of illness and health may lack the necessary basis for understanding what kind of a responsibility it is that they are supposed to assume.

Criticism of the self-care concept is not new. It can be encountered in a number of places – for example, among psychologists and nurses who are today part of the team around the diabetes patient. These people have subscribed to the concept of empowerment, which in this context means that the health professionals help the patients to discover and use their inherent abilities and resources in order to master their diabetes.

Having adopted empowerment, the health professionals are obliged to accept the patient's agenda and ask questions concerning the patient's worries and choices. At the same time, they must support the patient with ongoing teaching throughout the entire process. Lack of success with, for instance, lifestyle changes, must be turned from being a personal failure, in which one has not managed one's self-care satisfactorily – thereby getting a bad conscience and a sense of guilt – into being an experience that can be used positively in the future. This involves a complete change of paradigm, in which we give up the idea that "the patients must do as we say" (compliance) and to a higher degree accept the patient's own resources and choices (empowerment).

Empowerment may be the way forward, but a number of researchers ask, however, whether the health professionals have not simply adopted empowerment without having realized the consequences for the Health Service, themselves and the patients. Studies have shown that patients experience an absence of self-determination and acceptance despite the fact that the health personnel themselves believe that they are promoting empowerment. The new approach to health education is not yet fully integrated in the interdisciplinary diabetes team.

The political responsibility

In the interdisciplinary cooperation, it is our intention that the patient should be at the centre of the treatment, but the treatment is often fragmented into two or more processes rather than being a coordinated interdisciplinary process. As the Danish Health Service is organized today, with, for example, the responsibility for the treatment of type 2 diabetes chiefly being in general practice, the general practitioner rarely has the possibility of offering and coordinating longer-lasting courses of treatment and teaching that are adapted to the patient's needs and resources. Depending on where in the country the doctor practises, the patient can be referred to, for instance, "exercise on prescription" or dietician guidance, but a systematic coordination based on the patient's agenda and resources, and thereby possibilities for optimal self-care, is probably a rare occurrence. The good processes also encounter difficulties in the interfaces both between the primary and secondary sectors and between the health and social services. The development from paternalism to self-care has left resource-weak patients in the lurch. At the same time, there can be no doubt that the intention of wanting the best for the patients has always been present – also in Hagedorn's days.

In the light of history, we can see that the Health Service has to some degree been fighting an unequal struggle against the development of an unhealthy Western lifestyle. The trend towards a fattier diet and less exercise has been of great importance for the increased incidence of diabetes, but politicians hesitate to introduce measures that can promote self-care in connection with buying food, for instance by exempting healthy foodstuffs from VAT and ensuring healthy food in schools and canteens, or actually making very fatty and sugary food illegal in these places. Such a laissez-faire attitude seems quite inexplicable in a modern society like Denmark. It is interesting that society today can be paternalistic when it is a matter of obligatory seatbelts or banning smoking, and yet cannot get around to stimulating self-care by making healthy choices easier. Politicians have a range of management tools to be used, for instance, in cooperation with urban planners and others to make it necessary for us to get more exercise on a daily basis by introducing more car-free zones, establishing cycle paths and increasing the number of gym lessons at school. It is as if society's obligation is occasionally restricted to individual self-care and voluntary initiatives despite the fact that national programme declarations and strategies for public health emphasize the shared – and little wished for – paternalistic common responsibility.

The right balance

We have described the development from paternalism to self-care in the field of diabetes. Perhaps today the pendulum swings too far towards self-care, making it mandatory. The future challenge will be to create a balance between a responsible paternalism ("coaching") based on professional experience and an education that comprises knowledge of the biological factors that make it so difficult to imitate the natural plasma insulin's variations on the one hand and self-care that is adapted to the individual's resources on the other. The balance must be created in cooperation between the interdisciplinary diabetes team, the Health Service across sectors and regions and the new municipalities in Denmark. But this is a heavy health professional and health educational task that the diabetes team cannot manage alone. It is also incumbent on politicians, administrators, institutions and workplaces to use the modern management tools in order to form society in such a way that self-care and healthy choices become easier for all.

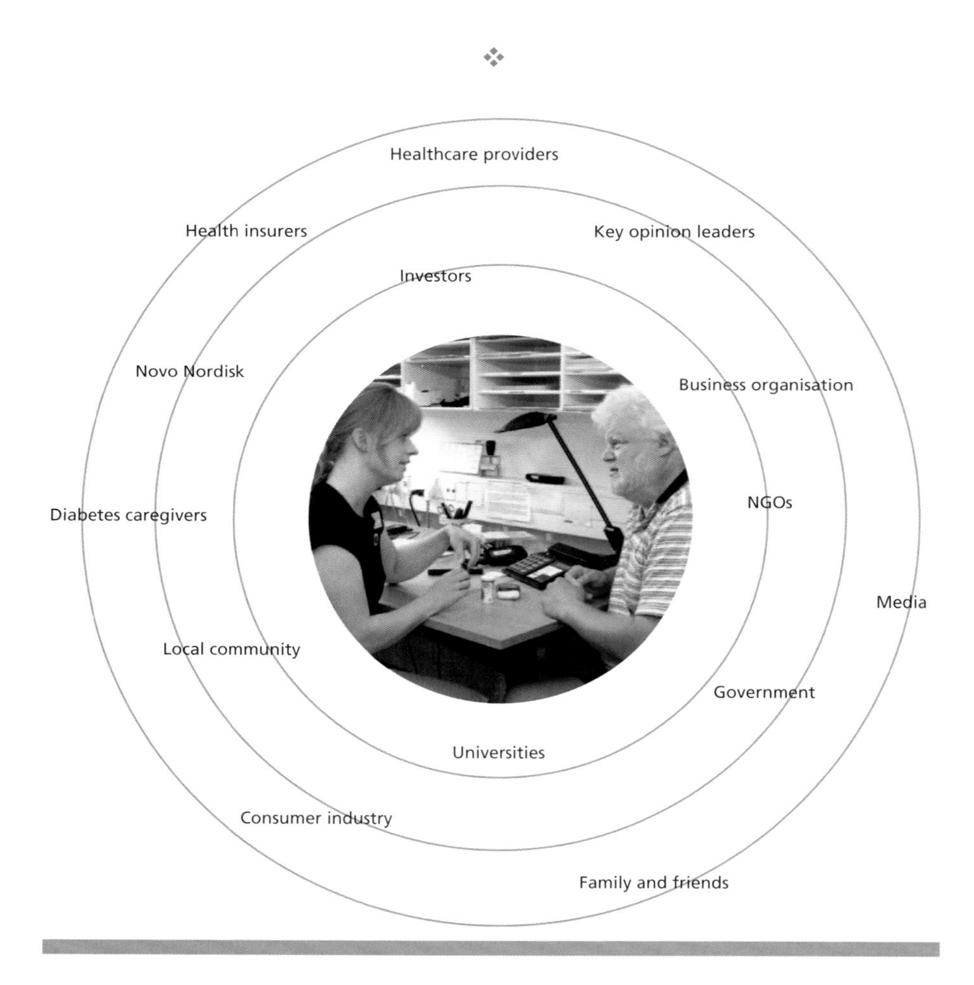

Patient and health care professional at the centre of all the factors that describe the complexity of diabetes treatment.
(From the DAWN Study).

SUPPLEMENTARY READING

Anderson RM, Funnell MM. Patient empowerment: reflections on the challenge of fostering the adoption of a new paradigm. Patient Educ Couns 2005;57:153-7.

Dørfler L, Hansen HP. Self-care – en litteraturbaseret udredning af begrebet. Copenhagen: Sundhedsstyrelsen, 2005.

Vallgårda S. Hvad er sundhedsfremme? En analyse af begrebet and styringsmetoderne. Tidsskrift for Forskning i Sygdom and Samfund 2005;3:15-31.

Haidet P, Kroll TL, Sharf BF. The complexity of patient participation: Lessons learned from patients' illness narratives. Patient Educ Couns 2006;62:323-9.

Paterson B. Myth of empowerment in chronic illness. J Adv Nurs 2001;34:574-81.

Wilson PM. A policy analysis of the expert patient in the United Kingdom: self-care as an expression of pastoral power? Health Soc Care Community 2001;9:134-42.

Williams G, Pickup JC. Textbook of Diabetes. 3rd ed. 2003, chapters 68-71.

ORGANIZATION OF DIABETES CARE IN DENMARK

ALLAN FLYVBJERG

Introduction

There is, at the present time, much focus on the treatment of persons with chronic diseases and on the active involvement of patients in dealing with their own disease. Concepts such as "coherent patient process", "self-care" and "uniform quality of treatment" have become key words for the government, the National Board of Health and a number of interest organizations. However, these concepts have been on the political agenda for diabetes for many years. Experiences from the field of diabetes function to a large degree as a model for a number of other chronic diseases.

There are nevertheless still a great number of unsolved problems concerning the treatment of both type 1 and type 2 diabetes. These are, for example, the constantly increasing number of persons with diabetes, a continued geographical imbalance in quality of treatment, an at times unclear division of labour between the primary and the secondary sectors, and an unacceptably large number of undiagnosed type 2 diabetes patients. Thus, new figures from the Danish National Board of Health show that today there are 220,000 diagnosed diabetes patients, of whom 20,000 have type 1 and 200,000 type 2 diabetes. Up to 200,000 patients with type 2 diabetes have not yet been diagnosed.

This chapter takes a look at some of the experience gained from the field of diabetes in Denmark over the past 75 years. There is no doubt that the credit for the advances that have been made in this field must be shared among many people. We have a very long tradition in Denmark of research into and treatment of diabetes and related late complications. A Danish insulin production that started only one year after the discovery in Toronto gave early high quality to the treatment. HC Hagedorn's establishment of Steno Memorial Hospital, Denmark's first diabetes hospital, 75 years ago has since been of great importance for diabetes treatment. Finally, the Diabetes Association's many years of work for the country's diabetes patients has been a cornerstone in Danish diabetes care.

Mileposts in diabetes care in Denmark

Centring on the work of the Diabetes Association, the present chapter reviews a series of events that are considered to have been of major importance for diabetes care in Denmark. The Diabetes Association's long tradition of care and information for those with diabetes and their relations has undoubtedly made a major contribution to the advances that have today been made in the field. Furthermore, in its constructive interaction with both health professionals and many voluntary workers the Diabetes Association has exercised a strong political influence.

The Danish Diabetes Association is founded

1940 was a landmark year for Nils Jørgensen and Axel Nielsen. They had been admitted to Hvidøre Diabetes Sanatorium in Klampenborg because of their diabetes. At Hvidøre, they were deeply moved by the many children who were admitted with diabetes. The thought that these children were facing a future with diabetes as their companion for the rest of their lives inspired them to do something. On Thursday, 12 December 1940, an important step was taken. Together with 72 others, they held the found-

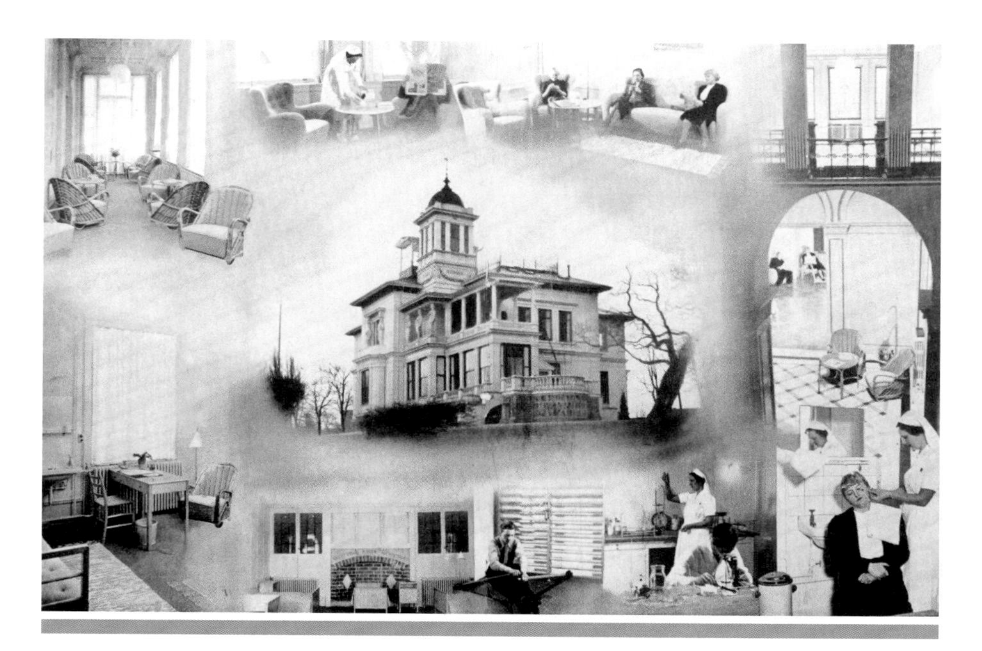

During a stay in 1940 at the manor-like Hvidøre Diabetes Sanatorium, Niels Jørgensen and Axel Nielsen conceived the idea of an association for diabetes patients.

ing general meeting in the National Association of Diabetics. The Danish Diabetes Association was thus established a few years after the diabetes associations in England and Australia, the same year as the American association, and several years before the other Scandinavian associations.

1940 was a difficult time at which to start a national association. Denmark was under German occupation, and funding was scarce. Nevertheless, it proved possible to build up an administration, local branches and much else. Only four months after the founding of the Association, the first bulletin for members made its appearance but this was possible only because the founders of the Association themselves donated money to it. From the start, the Association's activities were met with great sympathy and understanding among the population, among politicians and also among the medical profession. As an illustration of this broad acceptance of the Diabetes Association, the chairman Nils Jørgensen writes in the preface to one of the Association's first books from 1943 [1]: "*Despite its youth, the National Association of Diabetics has already carried out a number of tasks of a valuable nature for diabetics who are in difficult circumstances and for their homes. What strongly confirms the justification of starting the National Association is the encouraging understanding the Association has encountered from the press, the radio, medical circles and all sections of society. Especially the press has followed the National Association's work with keen interest and through innumerable articles helped to make easier the fulfilment of the National Association's tasks at the same time as an interest in the circumstances of thousands who are suffering from diabetes has been awoken*".

Early focus on care and self-care

Despite a difficult start, the Diabetes Association's economy was consolidated, and it became an inviolable principle to administer the Association's money with care and consideration for the needs the Diabetes Association was intended to cover. Right from the start, care and information were very central goals. Soon it became possible to establish a supporting foundation for needy members so that no one should be without the opportunity to have a stay at the diabetes hospitals of that time, Steno Memorial Hospital and Hvidøre Diabetes Sanatorium. Furthermore, a foundation was established for work with children with diabetes, so that the children could take part in holiday camps together with other children with diabetes.

Already in 1943, three years after it was founded, the Association published its first guidelines for patients [1]. In the foreword to the book, the chairman Nils Jørgensen writes: "*For diabetes patients and their relatives, it is of the greatest importance to have a detailed knowledge of both the disease and its treatment, and this is a field that, however much he would like to, the general practitioner cannot manage because of lack of time."*

In the preface to the same publication, district medical officer Johan Kaas writes: "*All patients have a certain right to know about the diseases they are suffering from, and this particularly applies to the protracted diseases. There has long been a need for a Danish popular description of diabetes, its characteristics and its treatment. We must therefore be grateful to the National Association of Diabetics for its initiative in presenting such a description. The present book is sufficiently exhaustive without being too broad, and it is pleasantly free of technical loan words and medical Latin. I believe that all diabetes patients will derive much benefit from reading the book, and when they have read it, they should keep it close at hand so that they can turn to it as to a good friend when there is some question about their disease that causes them difficulty.*"

That the Diabetes Association's early publication in support of self-care was in itself an epoch-making initiative can be illustrated by the fact that a publication from the National Board of Health from 2006 on self-care [2]

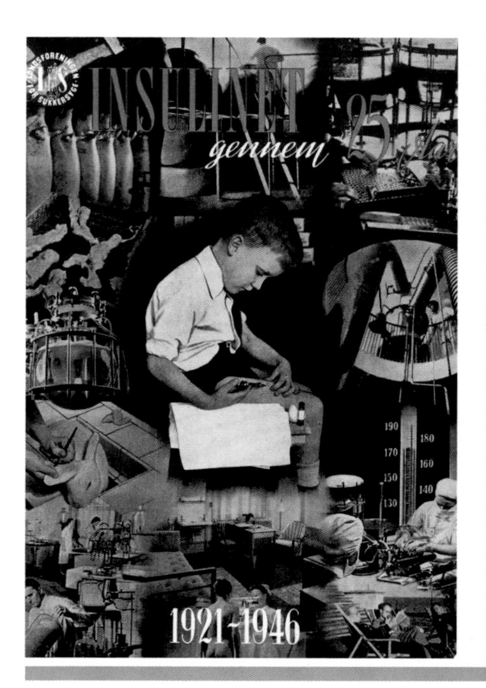

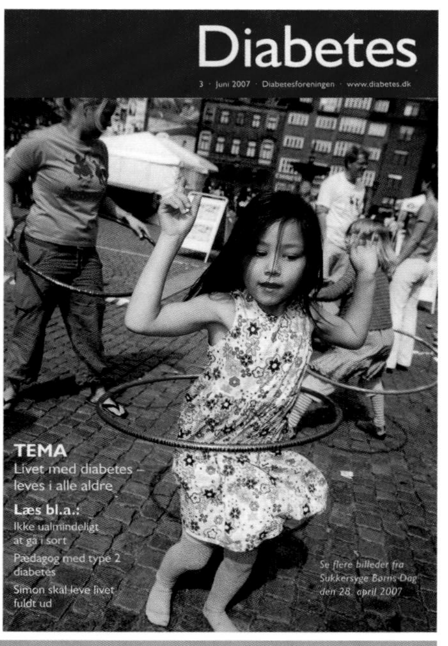

From order and discipline to free creativity. Title sheets from the Danish Diabetes Association's publications in 1946 and 2007 respectively.

states: "*The patient's self-care and the Health Service's support of it are a cardinal point, and this report focuses on the possibilities of involving the patient as an active participant in the monitoring and treatment of his or her disease*".

Information campaigns, support for research and international cooperation are initiated

From initially having been founded chiefly to help children with diabetes, the Diabetes Association gradually expanded its activities. Under its chairman Dr Alfred Hey's leadership, the period 1953-1973 was characterized by many nationwide information campaigns, which received strong backing in most major towns. The information work now extended to include doctors and nurses who had a need to learn about the treatment of diabetes and the needs people with diabetes had. Meetings for doctors were held in Nyborg as part of the work to increase the cooperation between general practitioners, specialists, hospitals and the Diabetes Association [3]. In agreement and collaboration with the Diabetes Association's medical council headed by Professor Niels B Krarup, a consensus matured for a substantial increase in the Association's support for scientific research. From a total of DKK 600 in 1950, the sum rose to DKK 25,000 in 1965, when the Diabetes Association's 25th anniversary was marked by a meeting in Domus Medica in Copenhagen in which representatives of the National Board of Health and of other public authorities participated. Since then, support for research and development from the Diabetes Association has steadily increased and today amounts to about DKK 5 million per year.

The international diabetes work started in 1949, when the first international diabetes congress was held in Brussels. Denmark was represented in a committee comprising all the participating countries by Professor Erik Warburg and the Diabetes Association's chairman Nils Jørgensen. In 1952, a corresponding congress was held in Leiden, Holland, with the participation of 20 countries [3]. From these modest beginnings emerged the International Diabetes Federation (IDF), which today numbers 200 diabetes associations in 158 countries, and which holds a world congress every third year.

At the international congress in Holland, the idea arose among the participants from the Scandinavian countries that it could be useful to establish a Scandinavian diabetes network. In connection with the Diabetes Association's representative assembly in Copenhagen in 1952, the "Nordic Diabetic's Cooperation Committee" was established with Nils Jørgensen as chairman. The committee immediately embarked on the practical work, and a number of organizational matters of common interest were handled.

Many topics were discussed, among other things, ways of helping to find increased support for research into diabetes and the occupational problems facing diabetes patients [3]. This cooperation has developed over the years and is still vigorously alive to this very day with annual meetings in Scandinavia.

Long-term political strategy initiated

In 1973, Alfred Hey wished to be replaced after 20 years as chairman for the Diabetes Association. Rehabilitation director Sven A Hellesen took over the post in the period 1973-1983, and drawing on his highly developed organizational insight and skills, he began a fairly radical restructuring of the Association and its work both internally and externally. This proved to be the beginning of better cooperation in connection with diabetes treatment. In close collaboration with the Diabetes Association's medical council, which now had chief physician Torsten Deckert as its chairman, the Association took an important step that would contribute to promoting cooperation among diabetes-engaged doctors, nurses, dieticians, podiatrists and social counsellors [3]. The general question of the Organisation of diabetes treatment in Denmark' was placed on the political agenda in the hope that it would be possible to establish an interdisciplinary coordination of the treatment of persons with diabetes.

In spring 1977, the Diabetes Association held an introductory meeting on the subject, and the participants in this meeting were a circle of diabetes doctors, nurses, dieticians, etc. all with detailed knowledge of the circumstances of diabetes patients. A working group was set up at the meeting with chief physician Anders Frøland as chairman. The group's report, which outlined a number of proposals for the improvement of diabetes treatment, was sent to the National Board of Health and to the county authorities. The report also formed the foundation for a seminar in 1979, at which the main topic had to do with *"Health educational challenges in diabetes treatment"*. Concepts such as "the establishment of specialist teams in each county" and "uniform guidelines for diabetes treatment" saw the light of day for the first time.

Two important reports on the organization of diabetes treatment

In 1980, as a result of the Diabetes Association's increasing political lobbyism and influence, the National Board of Health set up a committee to discuss the question of the organization of diabetes treatment in Denmark. In 1981, the National Board of Health thus published the report: "Diabetes. Organization of Research and Treatment" (known as "The Red Report" –

after the colour of the cover) [4]. In this report, it was proposed that in each county one or more centres for diabetes treatment should be established, typically attached to a medical department headed by a consultant with a strong interest in diabetes. These centres were also to be staffed by nurses, dieticians, and podiatrists specializing in diabetes. This proposal was fiercely supported by the Diabetes Association at hearings and negotiations all across the country. Consultant Anders Frøland was a major driving force in this work during his period as chairman from 1983 to 1990. The good intentions of the report received very varied backing in the county councils. For years after the publication of the report, one could observe significant qualitative and quantitative differences in diabetes treatment throughout the country. Furthermore, the increasing number of persons with type 2 diabetes was a problem that *"The Red Report"* had not addressed satisfactorily. Under the influence of the Diabetes Association headed by Anders Frøland, and later Professor Carl Erik Mogensen as chairman in 1990–1994, it became clear that there was a need for an updating of the recommendations for both type 1 and type 2 diabetes. In 1991, the National Board of Health therefore set up a working group tasked with reassessing the treatment of patients with diabetes. Besides Anders Frøland and Carl Erik Mogensen, the group comprised a large number of other leading diabetes experts.

The report *"Diabetes treatment in Denmark – future organization"* was launched in 1994 and focused on five main areas [5]. Thus, the report recommended: the development of a national plan for diabetes care; that diabetes patients themselves should increasingly take care of their own disease; that diabetes outpatient clinics should be staffed by diabetes teams (doctors, nurses, clinical dieticians, podiatrists, so-

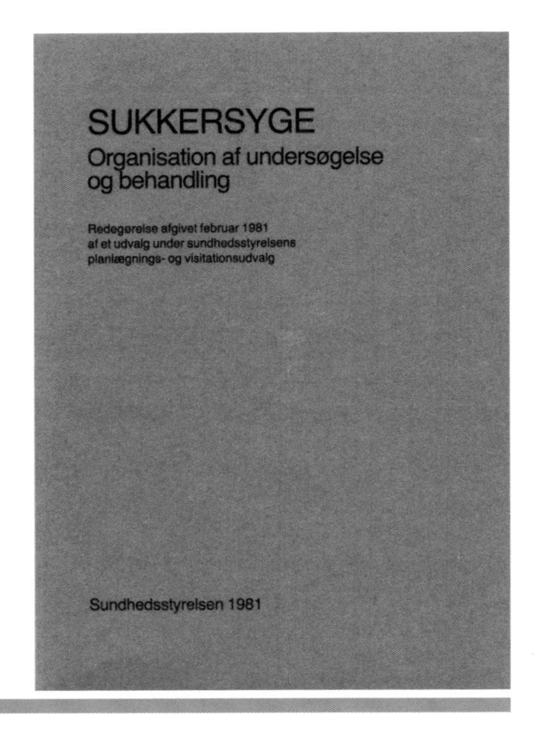

The Red Report, 1981. The state's first initiative to organize diabetes treatment in Denmark.

cial counsellors and with the possibility of psychologist assistance); and that country diabetes committees should be established in all the counties in Denmark with representation of diabetes patients [5]. At the same time, a broadly composed diabetes monitoring group was set up under the National Board of Health.

As was the case with "The Red Report", the intentions from the "1994 Report" were implemented with varying success in different places in the country. In a number of counties, diabetes treatment was entirely satisfactory, and in other counties there was considerable room for improvement. The problems linked with obtaining a uniform improvement of diabetes treatment were caused by, among other things, short-term book-keeping considerations about who was to foot the bill, the state, the county or the municipality. However, another contributory factor was that – despite good intentions on the part of the Danish Endocrine Society – it did not prove possible to establish a nationwide instrument for quality control. In the years following the publication of the report, the Diabetes Association worked hard to raise the quality of diabetes treatment in the counties that most lagged behind.

Increased focus on type 2 diabetes

Already in the drawing up of the National Board of Health's "1994 Report", a start was made on recommendations for the regulation and treatment of type 2 diabetes [5]. At that time, however, there was not sufficient knowledge concerning the natural history of the disease, and there was a lack of findings from large, well-controlled treatment studies. Up through the 1990s, there was, however, intense focus on the disease partly because of a pronounced rise in its incidence and because of figures indicating that up to 50 % of all type 2 cases were undiagnosed. The publication of the "United Kingdom Prospective Diabetes Study" (UKPDS) was of great importance for the treatment of type 2 diabetes abroad and in Denmark. Thus, in 2000, a number of leading diabetes experts published a Danish consensus report on the tracing and treatment of type 2 diabetes [6]. Under pressure from the Diabetes Association, it became more and more evident in Professor Oluf Borbye Pedersen's period as chairman from 1994 to 2000 that it was necessary to launch a targeted effort against type 2 diabetes. At the initiative of the Diabetes Association, the National Board of Health began a comprehensive medical technology assessment (MTV) collecting knowledge in the field of type 2 diabetes, a task that would take three years [7]. A large number of Denmark's leading diabetes experts took part in this work, and topics such as early detection of diabetes, early detection of late-diabetic complications, and pharmaceutical and non-pharmaceutical treatment were in focus [7].

In order to attract more political attention to the prevention and treatment of type 2 diabetes, the Diabetes Association held a conference at Christiansborg in autumn 2001 on "The organization of diabetes treatment in Denmark". Especially politicians, administrators and the chairpersons of the county diabetes committees were invited to this hearing. The conference was followed up by a nationwide campaign in 2002-2003 aimed at promoting the detection of undiagnosed diabetes among individuals at risk. During the same period, moreover, the Diabetes Association held hearings in all the counties inviting local politicians, health personnel and persons with diabetes to participate. The socio-economic aspects of diabetes had already been touched upon in the "1994 Report" [5], and it was these factors that were the main theme of the Diabetes Association's hearings. It was argued that a targeted effort against the development of late-diabetic complications would benefit both individuals with diabetes and the economy as a whole. During the IDF's World Congress in Paris in 2003, the Diabetes Association took the initiative and arranged one of the only seminars with this focus. The Diabetes Association received much commendation for this work.

National programme of action for diabetes

On 21 November 2003, came the great moment of release and the proof that the Diabetes Association's political work over so many years had borne fruit. The Minister of the Interior and Health Lars Løkke Rasmussen and the Diabetes Association jointly presented "the programme of action for diabetes" at a press conference at Christiansborg [8]. The target group for the programme of action comprised both type 1 and type 2 diabetes. At the same time, a broadly composed diabetes steering group was established under the auspices of the National Board of Health, with a proactive mandate [8]. Examples of concretely formulated tasks of an urgent nature were: monitoring and quality control of diabetes treatment, tracing of undiagnosed patients with type 2 diabetes, the issuing of updated guidelines for doctors and patients regarding type 2 diabetes, and a special effort directed towards pregnant diabetes patients. The work of establishing a Danish Diabetes Database (DDD) for both type 1 and type 2 diabetes was begun shortly after and the treatment of pregnant patients with diabetes was soon centralized at four large centres with high expertise. In 2004, moreover, all general practitioners in Denmark received updated and evidence-based guidelines for the tracing and treatment of type 2 diabetes [9]. Finally, in 2005, the Organisation of General Practitioners in Denmark drew up patient guidelines together with the Diabetes Association for type 2 diabetes, which could be distributed by general practitioners free of charge.

Diabetes treatment in the future

As appears from the aforementioned, the wish to establish "Coherent diabetes processes on the premises of the diabetes patient" and "Support of the patient's own resources" has for many years defined the objectives of the work to achieve better diabetes care in Denmark. Moreover, it seems clear that the objectives have not yet been fully met. It is therefore positive that the National Board of Health is at present systematically collecting the existing knowledge on the effect of self-monitoring, self-treatment and patient education in relation to a number of chronic diseases, among them type 1 and type 2 diabetes [2, 10]. It is also positive that the National Board of Health is engaged in describing the essential components of coherent process programmes [11, 12]. Thus, work is being done both on a description of a generic process programme for chronic disease, and on a specific process description for diabetes [11, 12]. The reports describe the necessary requirements for the health work, the organization of the work among different sectors in the health system, tools for stimulation of self-care and the implementation and monitoring of quality [11, 12]. The entry into force of the municipal reform in 2007 will undoubtedly affect the implementation of this work in both the regions and municipalities. It is to be hoped that the ongoing constructive and forward-looking initiatives for the establishment of a coherent diabetes process and supported self-care will receive the intense political attention that is required. The Diabetes Association will work to ensure that the necessary political measures prove to be sufficiently specific and binding to meet the documented needs of this field of public health – and not least of patients with diabetes.

Events and initiatives of importance for diabetes care in Denmark

1940	"The National Association of Diabetics" founded in Odense.
1965	The 25th anniversary of "The Diabetes Association" is marked by a major conference on diabetes in Copenhagen.
1977	The Diabetes Association begins long-term political work for better and more uniform diabetes treatment throughout the country.
1979	Working group under the Diabetes Association publishes a report with concrete proposals for improved organization of diabetes treatment.
1981	The National Board of Health publishes the report: "Diabetes: Organization of Research and Treatment (The Red Report)".
1994	The National Board of Health publishes the report: "Diabetes Treatment in Denmark: Future Organization (The 1994 Report)". The National Board of Health establishes a Diabetes Monitoring Group.
2000	The Danish Endocrine Society publishes a consensus report on type 2 diabetes.
2001	The Diabetes Association holds a conference at Christiansborg on "The organization of diabetes treatment".
2002	The Diabetes Association holds hearings in the counties throughout the country and launches a nationwide campaign for tracing type 2 diabetes among individuals at risk.
2003	The National Board of Health publishes the Medical Technology Assessment (MTV report) on type 2 diabetes.
2003	Together with the Diabetes Association, the Minister of Health launches the "Programme of Action for Diabetes". The National Board of Health sets up a Diabetes Control Group.
2004	The work of establishing the Danish Diabetes Database (DDD) is started.
2004	The Danish Society for General Medicine (DSAM) publishes an evidence-based guideline on the tracing and treatment of type 2 diabetes. At the same time, DSAM and the Diabetes Association jointly publish a patient guideline for type 2 diabetics.
2005	Inspired by experience from the field of diabetes, the National Board of Health issues a publication on organizational factors in the treatment of chronic disease.
2006	Inspired by experience from the field of diabetics, the National Board of Health issues an evidence-based report on "Self-monitoring, self-treatment and patient education in connection with chronic disease".
2007	The National Board of Health publishes the report "Process programme for diabetes".

REFERENCES

1. *Hey A. Sukkersyge: Hverdagens vejledning. Odense Amts Bogtrykkeri 1943*
2. *Patienten med kronisk sygdom: Selvmonitorering, egenbehandling og patientuddannelse. Sundhedsstyrelsen 2006*
3. *Jensen O. Fra tanke til handling. Diabetes (Tidsskrift for Sukkersyge) 1990;3:5-15*
4. *Sukkersyge: Organisation af undersøgelse og behandling. Sundhedsstyrelsen 1981*
5. *Diabetesbehandling i Denmark: fremtidig organisation. Sundhedsstyrelsen 1994*
6. *Beck-Nielsen H, Henriksen JE, Hermansen K, Madsen LD, de Fine Olivarius N, Mandrup-Poulsen T, Pedersen OB, Richelsen B, Schmitz O. Type 2 diabetes og det metaboliske syndrom – diagnostik og behandling. Klaringsrapport no. 6, 2000*
7. *Type 2 diabetes, medicinsk teknologivurdering af screening, diagnostik og behandling. Sundhedsstyrelsen og Center for Evaluering and Medicinsk Teknologivurdering 2003*
8. *Handlingsplan om diabetes. Indenrigs- and Sundhedsministeriet. 2003*
9. *Type 2-diabetes i almen praksis: En evidensbaseret vejledning. Dansk Selskab for Almen Medicin 2004*
10. *Kronisk sygdom – patient, sundhedsvæsen og samfund. Forudsætninger for det gode patientforløb. Sundhedsstyrelsen 2005*
11. *Forløbsprogram for diabetes. Sundhedsstyrelsen 2007*
12. *Forløbsprogram for kronisk sygdom. Sundhedsstyrelsen 2007*

INSULIN RESISTANCE – A STORY OF THE BIRTH OF A CONCEPT

HENNING BECK-NIELSEN

Introduction

The story of the concept of insulin resistance is relatively short and closely linked with the story of the discovery of the insulin receptor and the description of type 2 diabetes as an independent disease. A story in which Denmark has played a role, and a story that I myself have experienced and am a part of, but also a story about a number of visionary doctors and researchers.

The discovery of insulin took place 50 years before the discovery of the insulin receptor. Until 1970, almost all focus in diabetes research was therefore on insulin secretion, especially in relation to type 1 diabetes. It was therefore also natural to take an interest in the beta-cell function in patients with type 2 diabetes. The investigation of this disease stood, so to speak, on the shoulders of type 1 diabetes. And, indeed, the first pharmacological treatment was directed at the beta-cells, when sulfonylureas were launched for the stimulation of insulin secretion in 1955. However, there were no or only few researchers who prior to 1971 discussed insulin's effect at the cellular level. The effect on glucose transport, glycogen synthesis and glucose oxidation was known, but before 1971, no one had any idea as to how insulin affected the intracellular metabolism.

My diabetes teacher at the medical school in Århus was Professor Knud Lundbæk, who explained to us curious students that insulin could not penetrate into the cell – it sat outside and waved to the enzymes.

Knud Lundbæk, who at this time was one of the world's most well-known diabetologists, was very charismatic and a major figure in diabetes research in Denmark – one listened to him. In Århus, he built up a model endocrinological department, where research and clinical practice went hand in hand.

However, without any special publicity, a medical endocrinological department was established at Århus County Hospital, also with diabetology as a speciality. Here, another type of senior consultant was appointed, namely Niels Schwartz Sørensen, who came from Zealand and had both feet on the ground. He had worked his way up in the academic world through stays at various institutions among others the Steno Memorial Hospital, where under the expert guidance of Thomas Rosenberg, he had written his doctoral thesis on phosphorylases in the liver. Niels Schwartz Sørensen understood better than most the metabolism of glucose and fat. Thus, he held the view that an understanding of the metabolism of the fat could be the way to an understanding of type 2 diabetes – a hypothesis that later proved to be visionary.

The insulin receptor

In 1971, something happened that changed the history of diabetes just as significantly as the discovery of insulin had done in 1921 – the discovery of the insulin receptor. A French researcher by the name of Pierre Freychet and his mentor Jesse Roth published the first work showing that insulin is bound specifically to the cell membrane [1].

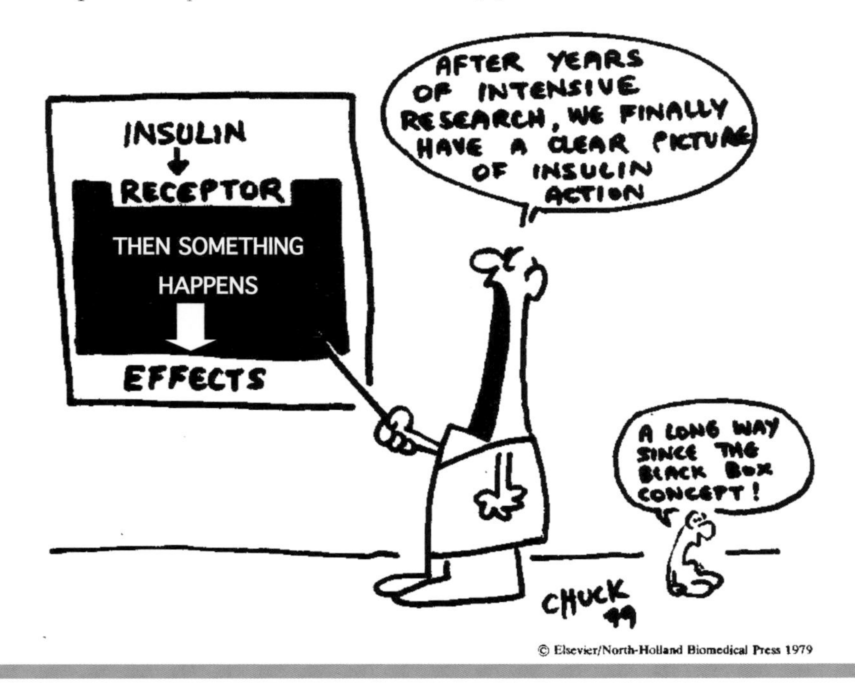

A perceptive artist's (Pierre De Meyts) mocking view of the insulin receptor and its effects in the year 1979.

The place of binding quickly turned out to be a characteristic anatomical structure, namely the insulin receptor, which can specifically bind insulin and only exceptionally other hormones and in such cases with much lower affinity. In this way, it had been clarified how a cell discriminates among the many hormones that pass its surface, and how through binding to the insulin receptor insulin can regulate the intracellular metabolism. Lundbæk had been right that insulin does not penetrate into the cell, but attaches itself to the receptor and waves to the enzymes. The discovery of the insulin receptor was of enormous importance for the understanding of the way in which insulin works, for the understanding of the concept of insulin resistance and for the treatment of type 2 diabetes. To me, it is surprising that this epoch-making discovery has not – yet – been awarded a Nobel Prize.

In 1974, Niels Schwartz Sørensen went to a congress in Belgium, where he chose to listen to Jesse Roth's lecture on the new discovery, the insulin receptor. Back in the department at Århus County Hospital, Niels Schwartz Sørensen had just hired two new, young registrars with a thirst for research, who met outside his door on 1 April 1974. The young doctors were Oluf Pedersen and the present writer, Henning Beck-Nielsen. Shortly after our appointment as clinical registrars, Niels Schwartz Sørensen presented us with the idea that we should study the insulin receptor, as it was obvious for him that insulin's effect at the cellular level was a regulated process, and that there could of course be defects at this level.

A heretical idea in many people's opinion!

Oluf Pedersen and I initiated a collaboration that later proved to be very fruitful. I was the first to be allowed to leave the clinic in order, as a clinical assistant, to start up the studies in the "research basement" under Århus County Hospital. The first task was to set up a human assay for the measurement of insulin receptors. It was not at this time possible to isolate human fat, muscle or liver – the three target tissues for insulin's effect. Fortunately, methods with lymphocytes had already been published. We chose to refine the methods and therefore studied monocytes. Niels Schwartz Sørensen, Oluf Pedersen and I paid a visit to Jesse Roth and Ronald Kahn's laboratories at NIH to learn the secrets and experienced here that a certain creativity was necessary to interpret the tricky binding curves. We also visited Associate Professor Jørgen Gliemann at the University of Copenhagen, who was already working with the binding of insulin to rat fat cells. The collaboration described above was of crucial importance for the start of the insulin receptor era at Århus County Hospital. With the monocyte as a model, we described the human insulin receptor for the first time in Denmark and probably in Europe too [2]. The news of this also reached Århus Municipal Hospital, but in the first instance did not lead to a closer collaboration between the two diabetes departments, though with one exception. We did establish good cooperation with Hans Ørskov, who was head of the "research basement" in Department M, Århus Municipal Hospital. Hans Ørskov could measure insulin. We needed that as we could not get the method to function ourselves. To most people's surprise, these measures showed that some diabetes patients had too much insulin in the blood and not as expected insulinopenia – a deficiency of insulin.

Our studies of the human insulin receptor soon became known, and a number of researchers visited the "research basement" at Århus County Hospital, among others Novo's director of research, Lise Heding, who came to see the new phenomenon with her own eyes. And at last, one morning when I was sitting in the outpatient clinic, came the call that was the accolade that confirmed my admission to the circle of researchers. Knud Lundbæk rang: *"If you'd like to tell us a little about the insulin receptor, I'll stand you a sandwich and a beer"*

The ice had been broken, and a new era had begun!

The clinical importance of the discovery of the insulin receptor

One cannot survive if one is born without insulin receptors, and severe genetic effects lead to severe insulin resistance, which is today called type A insulin resistance. Slightly disappointingly, not least in relation to our own expectations, it has not been possible to find, beyond a decrease in the number of insulin receptors, significant functional changes in the large group of patients with type 2 diabetes. This does not mean that there are not defects, besides the aforementioned type A defects that can cause insulin resistance and diabetes. For instance, it has turned out that one can form antibodies against one's own insulin receptor. Oluf Pedersen and I described one of the first cases of this kind in the literature in 1980 [3]. This form of insulin resistance is today called type B insulin resistance. At Department M, Odense University Hospital, we have described an entirely new disease, namely "hyperinsulinemic hypoglycaemia linked to a mutation in the human insulin receptor gene" – in everyday speech called "Morbus Olsen" after the name of the family that was first diagnosed [4]. This is a family with hypoglycaemia so severe that it can trigger cramps and unconsciousness, and it therefore led – also for the index person – to the erroneous diagnosis of epilepsy. "Morbus Olsen" is characterized by very high fixed serum insulin values around 1-5000 pmol/l, which we found were due to a mutation in the insulin receptor gene corresponding to the part of the molecule that accounts for the internalization of insulin, i.e. its degradation. The defect means that insulin is not degraded and therefore accumulates. The disease has proved to be dominant hereditary.

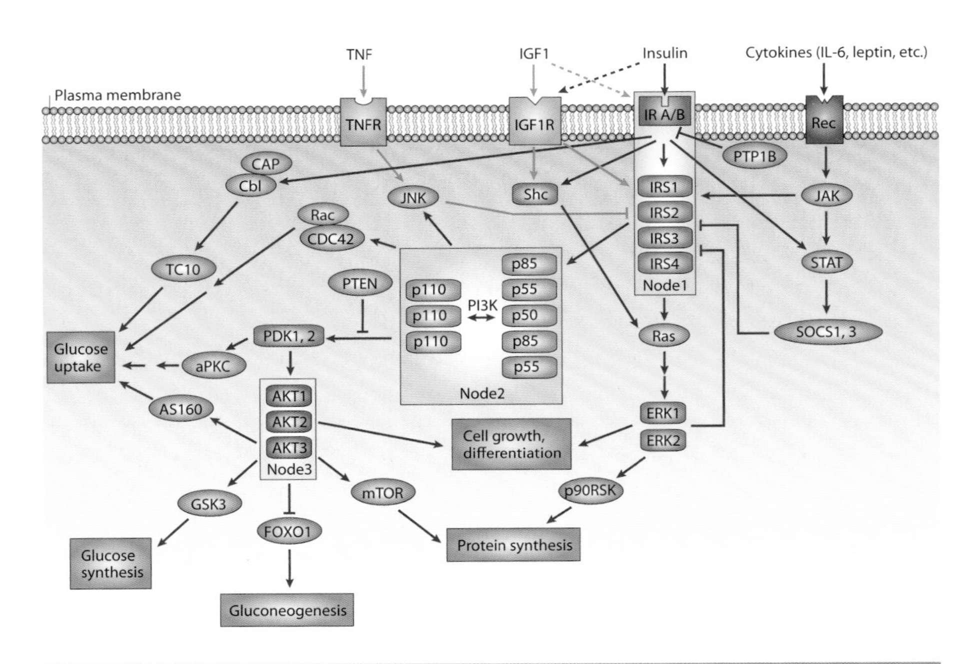

The art develops: To the right insulin signalling in 1981 and above as it is seen in 2006 (above). (Ugeskrift for Læger, 1981, and Nature Reviews, Molecular Cell Biology, 2006)

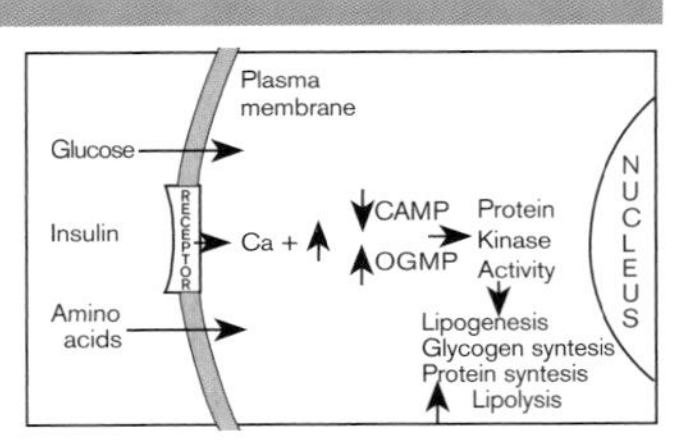

It can be treated with the hormone somatostatin. This hormone is sold as a pharmaceutical, and with this hormone, it has proved possible to keep persons with the disease, which has now been diagnosed in both England and China, free of symptoms.

The link between the insulin receptor and insulin effect

Even though the insulin receptor in itself cannot tell us why patients with type 2 diabetes are insulin resistant, the discovery opened the way to an understanding of how insulin works and an understanding of intracellular defects in the insulin-mediated glucose disposal.

Figure 1 shows three stages in the understanding of the mechanism by which insulin works since the discovery of the insulin receptor and up to today.

Insulin resistance – a new concept

With my point of departure in the clinic, my interest has constantly revolved around how these new discoveries could be used for the understanding of type 2 diabetes. The key to this understanding has proved to be an understanding of the concept of insulin resistance. When we began in 1974, this concept did not exist, except for the fact that a reduced insulin effect had been described in a number of patients with type 1 diabetes with antibodies against porcine insulin. The concept of insulin resistance can best be defined as "a reduced biological effect of insulin on the cellular metabolism, reduced in relation to the effect observed in 'normal' persons". The concept of insulin resistance, as it is defined above, was first introduced by Professor Gerald Reaven in the mid-1970s [5]. Reaven rediscovered insulin resistance at a time when the world could understand it thanks to the discovery of the insulin receptor, and that was his luck/ability. I still remember how when first reading about the concept, I thought this could be the start of a completely new era, but did not realize that my career would lie in this field. However, my intuition was correct. Today, insulin resistance is central to the understanding not only of type 2 diabetes, but also of cardiovascular diseases.

We developed a test – the insulin tolerance test – for the measurement of insulin sensitivity *in vivo*. With this test, we could show that obese persons with and without type 2 diabetes were insulin resistant, and we were also the first to show that a reduction of the calorie intake increased insulin sensitivity [6]. This is an insight that has been repeatedly confirmed and has formed the background for comprehensive intervention studies that have now shown with certainty that one can reduce the risk of developing type 2 diabetes, and that calorie restriction is an effective treatment of this disease. The insulin tolerance test has its limitations, and therefore, as the first in Europe to do so, we introduced the test that is today the gold standard, namely the hyperinsulinemic euglycemic clamp technique, through which the blood glucose concentration is kept constant through infusion of insulin and glucose. Fairly soon after, we also started up with muscle biopsies, which gave access to human muscle tissue for the first time in Denmark. At the same time, Oluf Pedersen had introduced the first Danish analysis for measurement of insulin binding to isolated human fat cells. We now had access to two of the three human target tissues for insulin, namely fat and muscle, while ethical considerations meant that the liver was still out of reach.

The USA

A wish to achieve a better understanding of the role of the muscles in the development of insulin resistance in type 2 diabetes led to a stay in San Diego, USA, with Professor Jerry Olefsky. Here I was introduced to Larry Mandarino. With Larry Mandarino as the main actor, we developed the method that more than any other has formed the backbone internationally in the investigation of the effect of insulin *in vivo* in humans, both in organs and at cellular level. The idea is to combine the clamp test infusion of radioactively marked glucose for measurement of the general glucose turnover and the liver's glucose production with indirect calorimetry for measurement of glucose and fat oxidation together with muscle biopsies to investigate the intracellular effect of insulin in the skeletal musculature. In this way, it is possible to set up dose response curves for the effect of whole-body glucose oxidation, fat oxidation and the liver's glucose oxidation (HGP) along with the dose response curve to the glucose and fat metabolism intracellularily in the skeletal musculature. This method applied to normal persons was published in the Journal of Clinical Investigation in 1987 [7]. That this was a pioneering work is underlined by the fact that at UCSD there was no calorimeter. However, we borrowed one from the State University of California, which was situated 15 km from San Diego. The calorimeter was larger than an American refrigerator (!), and on the day of the trial, we had to transport it from the State University to San Diego and back again. Transportation was by way of Larry Mandarino's Toyota van and was carried out by Larry Mandarino and the present writer. So don't say that research doesn't require muscles! On one of the trips, the rope tying the calorimeter to the Toyota came loose, and it was only thanks to a very swift reaction that it did not hit the tarmac. Had this happened, the already mentioned "high impact" article would never have seen the light of day, and my grant-financed stay would

A major finding in the author's research and in the understanding of insulin resistance: the absence of insulin-stimulating activation of the glycogen synthase in the skeletal muscles in patients with type 2 diabetes. The data represent mean ±SEM: a p<0.01 compared with control persons and b p<0,01 compared with persons with type 2 diabetes during insulin stimulation. (Beck-Nielsen, Diabetologia, 1991).

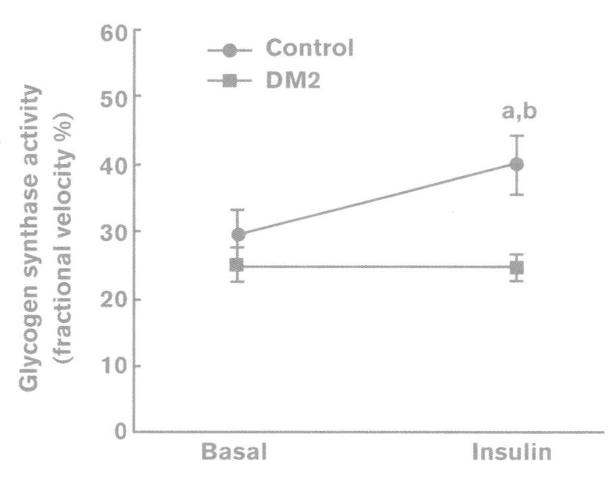

have undoubtedly come to a speedy end for economic reasons.

On arriving in San Diego, I was asked whether I could perform muscle biopsies, which I cheerfully said that I could (I had made a single attempt back home). One of the first trial persons was a volunteer, a former soldier from the war in Beirut, who had been standing in the second rank at the embassy explosion in the 1980s. He was very far from calm and complained loudly during the procedure, which might be surprising as he wore a green beret. This naturally made some people doubt my ability as a performer of biopsies, but the ultracentrifugation of his muscle tissue showed tens of thousand of microscopic metal particles from the bomb at the embassy. This explained his reaction and my problems in carrying out the biopsy. This story also shows how so-called normal controls can deviate from the expected, which may be the explanation for many strange scientific results over time in case-control studies.

I brought these methods home with me, and since then, they have been a treasured tool in many parts of the world and afforded many valuable results. Here I must mention our own discovery that glycogen synthase in the skeletal musculature of persons with type 2 diabetes cannot be stimulated with insulin, which together with Gerry Shulman's NM studies confirmed that peripheric insulin resistance is reduced insulin-mediated glycogen synthase [8].

The liver's glucose production (HGP)

One of the great advances with the new technology was that through the infusion of tritiated glucose in connection with the clamp, it became possible to study the liver's glucose production. That the liver plays an important role for glucose regulation has been known for a number of years, especially from animal experiments, but it was probably a surprise for most people that the first trials with the new technique *in vivo* in humans indicated that HGP was increased by 2-300 %. These results brought the focus to bear on the liver but later proved to have been seriously overestimated because of methodological errors. The estimate of the liver's glucose production was due to an incorrect use of the tracer technique, as Ole Hother-Nielsen and Diane Finegood from Los Angeles showed at an early stage [9]. Ole Hother-Nielsen has left a large fingerprint on research in this field, and his methods are now widely used all over the world. Studies with the new techniques have shown that in many patients with diabetes the liver's glucose production is normal or increased by at most 20 %. It has taken a very long time to get this message across. Science is often like a supertanker that is difficult to turn about, especially when the change of course may have consequences for one's funding. It is unfortunately typical that researchers find it hard to change their hypotheses, especially if it means that they have to reject earlier results. This is the case despite the fact that the falsification of one's own hypotheses ought to be a consecrated goal for researchers.

Insulin resistance in recent years

The history of insulin resistance will in the nature of things follow the trends that take place in science – one can say that they follow the "fashion". The available new techniques will often set the agenda, as will be described in the following by three examples.

In the last 30 years, in which insulin resistance has been studied more intensively, genetics has had a renaissance with the description of the genome. Twin studies in Odense based on the Danish Twin Register, the most complete in the world, soon showed that type 2 diabetes insulin resistance is not at all as hereditary as first assumed. Pernille Poulsen and Allan Vaag's studies also showed that for the main part, insulin resistance is due to environmental problems such as obesity and the intrauterine environment, while insulin secretion seems to have a large genetic component [10]. The history of the genetic field is, however, discussed elsewhere in this book.

Another field that has developed over the aforementioned 30-year period is the discovery of fat tissue as an endocrine organ that produces a number of peptides and hormones. I often think of all the supernatants from fat cells that we have thrown out in the course of the years without knowing that here lay the key to an understanding of insulin resistance. Even the discovery of the hormone adiponectin has proved crucial, as fat persons with large fat cells have reduced adiponectin secretion, which causes reduced insulin sensitivity in the liver and muscles. Among the first in the world to understand the endo- and paracrine effect of fat cells was Bjørn Richelsen, who in the old laboratory in the "research basement" of Århus County Hospital with great skill pursued Schwartz Sørensen's ideas about understanding fat cell metabolism as a tool for understanding insulin resistance and type 2 diabetes.

As already mentioned, the studies of insulin's effect in the skeletal musculature in patients with insulin resistance and type 2 diabetes have been helped along the way by the tradition for sports medicine that has characterized Denmark for many years, especially centred on the August Krogh Institute in Copenhagen. Basal studies of glycogen metabolism, glucose transport and, later, insulin signalling have been and are still an important precondition for many of the clinical studies performed among diabetes patients. Here special mention should be made of Jørgen Wojtaszewski and Kurt Højlund's studies of the insulin signalling cascade and the phosphorylation of glycogen synthase [11]. Through this, we shall probably achieve an understanding in the nearest future of why glycogen synthase cannot be activated by insulin in patients with type 2 diabetes.

The treatment of insulin resistance

As mentioned above, the last 40 years' research has mainly been of a pathophysiological nature, which has also given a good picture of why and how type 2 diabetes develops, but the great number of patients, which is increasing at the rate of 5 % annually, has together with the description of the disease meant that much more focus has been brought to bear on its treatment.

I remember that when I took part in my first scientific congress in Bergen in 1975, Professor Åkenes from Oslo said, freely quoted: "*Yet another congress without any clinical dividend*". This statement shocked me as I of course expected to come home with knowledge that I could use directly on our patients. However, it is not until recent decades that in a congress context, clinical research has been accepted on an equal footing with basic research. In the field of type 2 diabetes, UKPDS (the UK Prospective Diabetes Study) has indisputably been the turning-point. This very large study showed for the first time that it is worth treating type 2 diabetes intensively with pharmaceuticals. It also clarified three unresolved issues, showing: 1) that sulfonylurea did not cause cardiovascular death, which was a claim we had to live with for many years; 2) that insulin is not better in monotherapy than the peroral antidiabetics; and 3) that metformin is the only antidiabetic drug that can reduce the number of myocardial infarcts and reduce mortality, but only in overweight persons with type 2 diabetes. These results changed the treatment radically, so that today, metformin is the first-choice preparation. Furthermore, the study showed that multipharmacological treatment is necessary. The effects of the treatment were not, however, impressive and clearly showed that one cannot keep the HbA_{1c} value close to the normal area with monotherapy, as it increases gradually over the first year. The reason seems to be a rapid fall in the beta-cell function, which underscores that beta-cell preserving treatment must be the goal in the future, which can be achieved by, for example, concurrent treatment of the insulin resistance. Pharmacologically, however, this has only been possible in recent years with the introduction of the glitazones.

Summary and future developments

For me, and all those I have mentioned in this historical retrospect and undoubtedly also those I have not managed to name, it has been a fantastic experience to have been part of these 30 year's research into the insulin receptor, insulin resistance and type 2 diabetes and to experience in a short time that the investment in basic research has been able to yield such a swift and dramatic effect on practice in the clinic, where the prognosis for the disease has been significantly improved.

My account is heavily biased by the fact that I have been in the midst of it all, but this must be the intention behind this book, namely to be a personal account. This does not change the fact that Denmark has made its contribution. We are only one thousandth of the world's population, but produce one hundredth of the world's research. In respect of diabetes, the figure is probably closer to one tenth, especially if the impact of that research is taken into account.

Why has Denmark been able to play this role?

Some will hold the view that it is a matter of chance – and chance has often played a role – but there are also several persons who have a large part of the honour. In the story of insulin resistance and type 2 diabetes, Århus played a central role in the beginning, after which Copenhagen and Odense have made their presence felt. In Århus, this took place in the two "research basements", and, of course, it may seem symbolic that the research was consigned to the basement floor. For me, Niels Schwartz Sørensen's intuition and his interest in the fat cell have played an important role. Here we cannot speak of a strategic investment by a research council or a ministry – rather, on the contrary. The Research Council has, however, played a vital role. I remember from an early stage how great an encouragement it was for us the first time we received a grant from the Medical Research Council – a grant I have received without interruption ever since. Economically, it was important, but in terms of morale it was of incalculable importance. The doctoral thesis degree – now on its way out – played a very decisive role because as opposed to the PhD degree, it requires original research. It was a great impetus for the researchers of that time. The goal was good research. If successful it was also good for one's career. The PhD scheme today focus more on training researchers and less on original research. In addition to these two factors, Novo Nordisk has also played a major role for diabetes research in Denmark through the substantial economic support it has given to research and through its support to Steno Diabetes Center. This has helped to place Denmark on the world map. If diabetes is to maintain this position, it is important that original research is prioritized in research councils and foundations, that room is found for people with talent and initiative, and that the basic research at the universities is supported – the undergrowth is important.

People with passion and commitment who quickly saw the light and understood the importance of cooperation, not least internationally, are the explanation for this positive story about insulin resistance.

REFERENCES

1. *Freychet P, Roth J, Neville DM, Jr. Insulin receptors in the liver: specific binding of (125 I) insulin to the plasma membrane and its relation to insulin bioactivity. Proc Natl Acad Sci USA 1971;68:1833-7*
2. *Beck-Nielsen H. Insulin receptors in man. The monocyte as model for insulin receptor studies. Ugeskr Læger 1980;27:173-85*
3. *Pedersen O, Beck-Nielsen H, Heding L. Increased insulin receptors after exercise in patients with insulin-dependent diabetes mellitus. N Engl J Med 1980;302:886-92*
4. *Hojlund K, Hansen T, Lajer M, Henriksen JE, Levin K, Lindholm J, Pedersen O, Beck-Nielsen H. A novel syndrome of autosomal-dominant hyperinsulinemic hypoglycemia linked to a mutation in the human insulin receptor gene. Diabetes 2004;53:1592-8*
5. *Reaven GM. Banting lecture 1988. Role of insulin resistance in human disease. Diabetes 1988;37:1595-607*
6. *Beck-Nielsen H, Pedersen O, Sorensen NS. Effects of diet on the cellular insulin binding and the insulin sensitivity in young healthy subjects. Diabetologia 1978;15:289-96*
7. *Mandarino LJ, Wright KS, Verity LS, Nichols J, Bell JM, Kolterman OG, Beck-Nielsen H. Effects of insulin infusion on human skeletal muscle pyruvate dehydrogenase, phosphofructokinase, and glycogen synthase. Evidence for their role in oxidative and nonoxidative glucose metabolism. J Clin Invest 1987;80:655-63*
8. *Damsbo P, Vaag A, Hother-Nielsen O, Beck-Nielsen H. Reduced glycogen synthase activity in skeletal muscle from obese patients with and without type 2 (non-insulin-dependent) diabetes mellitus. Diabetologia 1991;34:239-45*
9. *Hother-Nielsen O, Beck-Nielsen H. Basal glucose metabolism in type 2 diabetes. A critical review. Diabetes Metab 1991;17:136-45*
10. *Vaag A, Henriksen JE, Madsbad S, Holm N, Beck-Nielsen H. Insulin secretion, insulin action, and hepatic glucose production in identical twins discordant for non-insulin-dependent diabetes mellitus. J Clin Invest 1995;95:690-8*
11. *Hojlund K, Staehr P, Hansen BF, Green KA, Hardie DG, Richter EA, Beck-Nielsen H, Wojteszewski JF. Increased phosphorylation of skeletal muscle glycogen synthase at NH2-terminal sites during physiological hyperinsulinemia in type 2 diabetes. Diabetes 2003;52:1393-402*
12. *Gaede P, Vedel P, Parving HH, Pedersen O. Elevated levels of plasma von Willebrand factor and the risk of macro- and microvascular disease in type 2 diabetic patients with microalbuminuria. Nephrol Dial Transplant 2001;16:2028-33*
13. *Poulsen MK, Henriksen JE, Hother-Nielsen O, Beck-Nielsen H. The combined effect of triple therapy with rosiglitazone, metformin, and insulin aspart in type 2 diabetic patients. Diabetes Care 2003;26:3273-9*

NOT MUCH AIR GUITAR
– TYPE 1 DIABETES GENETICS IN DENMARK

FLEMMING POCIOT

On 17 May 2000, under the heading *Not much air guitar*, the daily newspaper *Politiken* brought a 1½-page account of a small, informal meeting between diabetes researchers and geneticists from all around the world. There was no air guitar or smashed up furniture when on a weekend in April 2000 fifteen of the world's leading researchers met at the time-honoured Kokholm Hotel near Kandestederne in The Skaw. Nevertheless, the meeting would turn out to be a high point in international genetic research into type 1 diabetes. For some time, Jørn Nerup and I had been toying with the idea of a meeting at which some of the sharpest brains in the field would be assembled under informal circumstances, without tight agendas and without prearranged presentations. It had become clear that the final mapping of the genetics of type 1 diabetes would require extensive family material and therefore international cooperation. The Sehested Hansen Foundation made the necessary funds available, and we trusted that a meeting of this size under the right circumstances could deflate the otherwise large egos and stimulate discussion on new ideas, new ways of looking at things and even create a basis for collaboration rather than competition. We wanted the participants to "think outside the box", try out ideas and discuss them without reservations. Normally, there are not very good opportunities for this at congresses. The outcome of our meeting was an initiative that is unique in the field of genetic studies of multifactorial diseases. But more about this later. The Skaw meeting, as it is now called in type 1 diabetes circles, was the result of and the culmination to date of more than 25 years of genetic research into type 1 diabetes (T1D) at Steno Diabetes Center – previously Steno Memorial Hospital.

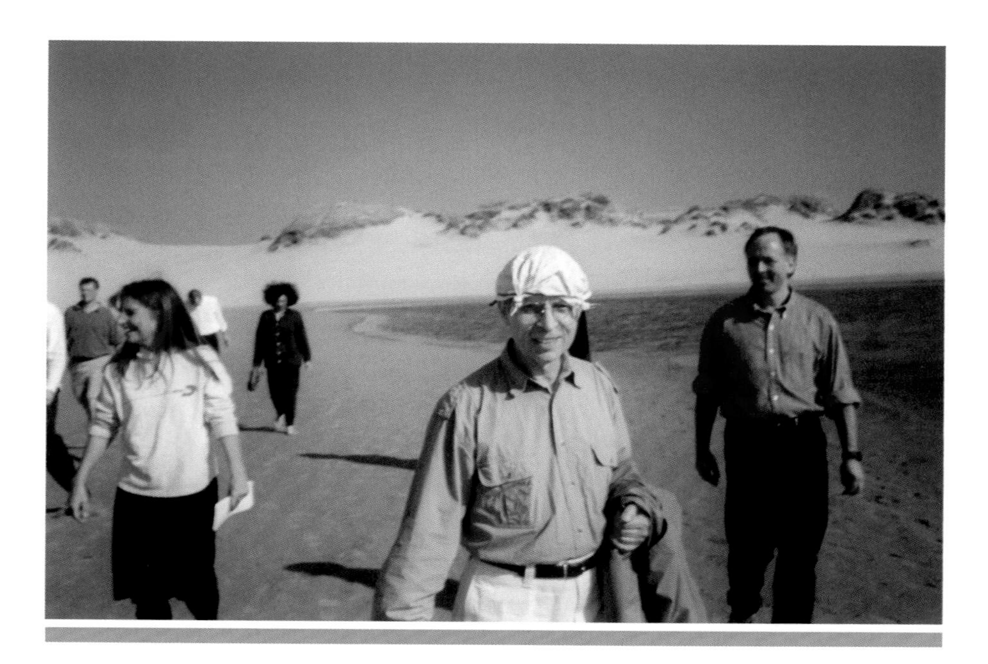

Some of the participants at the "Skaw Meeting" *during a break on a relaxed walk in Raabjerg Mile. In the picture, among others: Jürg Ott, Cecile Julier, Torben Hansen and the author (April 2000).* "Leading researchers they may be, but they're still a bunch of peculiar nerds", *as one of the accompanying family members observed.*

The pathogenetic and genetic identification of type 1 diabetes

It all began in 1974, when Nerup then at the County Hospital in Gentofte, together with colleagues from Frederiksberg Hospital, Bispebjerg Hospital, the Tissue Type Laboratory at Rigshospitalet and Morten Christy and Jacob E Poulsen from Steno Memorial Hospital, published the association between certain types of tissue (HLA antigens) and diabetes mellitus in the *Lancet* on 12 October 1974 [1]. This was an observation that had already been presented at the Scandinavian Diabetes Meeting the previous year. Prior to this, in 1971, Nerup and his colleagues had shown that diabetes in normal-weight, insulin-treated, young persons is a so-called autoimmune disease. This is in contrast to diabetes in obese, tablet- or diet-treated persons. These findings and the conclusion that from an immunological viewpoint, there are two pathogenetically different types of diabetes evoked quite a sensation, but were quickly confirmed by many other groups. Via a large number of animal experiments, Nerup pursued this observation and tried to explain it on the basis of 'molecular mimicry', in which immunogenic epitopes were common to the Coxsackie virus and a primary beta-cell antigen. Despite a comprehensive and exhaustive effort, it proved impossible to demonstrate the existence of this phenomenon. The negative result was surprising, unexpected and a threat to the hypothesis of autoimmunity from 1971. However, things quickly fell into place. Nerup got the idea that even though 'molecular mimicry' could not be proved, autoimmune insulin-requiring diabetes had to arise as the result of the interaction of one or more environmental factors with the patient's genetic "set-up", and that immune-response genes had to be involved. This led, as already mentioned, to the demonstration in 1974 of the association between HLA and insulin-requiring diabetes and the following hypothesis:

> *"... one or more immune-response genes associated with HL-A8 and/ or W15 might be responsible for an altered T-lymphocyte response. The genetically determined host response could fail to eliminate an infecting virus (Coxsackie B4 and others) which in turn might destroy the pancreatic beta-cells or trigger an autoimmune reaction against the infected organ ..."*

The authors found that certain serological HLA markers (HL-A8 and W15) exhibited strong disease association. Earlier works by Finkelstein et al. (1972) and Singal and Blajchman (1973) had suggested an association between HLA and diabetes, but because of what were probably technical problems, unambiguous results were not obtained. The *Lancet* work from 1974 is therefore the first that convincingly demonstrates an association between certain HLA markers and diabetes. Nerup et al. found moreover in this work that the association was strongest with a diabetes phenotype that was characterized by absolute insulin independence, early onset and normal weight. The work therefore also showed that with genetic markers it was possible to distinguish between the two main forms of diabetes, which at that time were designated as insulin-dependent (IDDM) and non-insulin-dependent diabetes mellitus (NIDDM). The authors write that they do not know how some HLA factors lead to an increased risk of insulin-dependent diabetes, and propose that genes in the HLA region other than those investigated in the article might also be of importance for the risk of disease. The *Lancet* study led to a long series of publications on HLA and diabetes from groups all around the world. A Medline search in 2007 produces more than 4,200 references to HLA and diabetes.

The HLA region makes up less than 0.15 % of our total genome, but is without doubt by far the best investigated. Traditionally, the HLA region is divided into three classes: class I, class II and class III. The article from

DRB1-DQB1		P/C Ratio
Haplotype 1	**Haplotype 2**	
03-0201	04-0302	18
04-0302	04-0302	13
01-0501	04-0302	6
03-0201	03-0201	5
04-0302	07-02	3
02-0602	x	0.015

HLA class II (DRB1-DQB1) genotypes listed according to type 1 diabetes-predisposition effect shown as patient/control (P/C) ratio. Note that the DR2-DQ6 haplotype gives pronounced protection.

1974 showed an association to diabetes of genes from the class I region. Subsequent studies soon showed that certain allele combinations from genes in class I, class II and class III are inherited far more frequently that one would expect, and more frequently than can be seen elsewhere in the genome. In other words, the region was characterized by pronounced linkage disequilibrium. This would prove to make the identification of the actual risk alleles a difficult matter. Although many groups soon focused on studies of HLA and diabetes, it was again groups around Jørn Nerup and Arne Svejgaard that in 1975 with Mogens Thomsen as first author showed that the association between insulin-requiring diabetes and HLA is primarily due to alleles in the class II region [2]. This is also the situation today: HLA class II alleles are those that primarily predispose to type 1 diabetes.

The development of new technology, among other things crystallographic studies, has taught us much about the function and structure of the genes in the HLA region, but even after 30 years' research, we have not yet obtained a full understanding of the association between HLA and T1D.

Further studies showed it to be probable that HLA class II alleles were neither sufficient nor necessary for the development of T1D. This means that other genes could also contribute to the genetic risk for T1D.

The discovery of the insulin genes

It was studies designed to reveal the inheritability of type 2 diabetes that would identify the next T1D gene. In 1980, Graeme Bell from Chicago in collaboration with, among others, David Owerbach had localized the human insulin gene to chromosome 11 and had furthermore demonstrated a number of sequence variations in the area. In 1981, Allan Permutt's group had suggested the possibility of an association between certain insulin gene sequence variations and non-insulin-requiring diabetes. David Owerbach came to Steno Memorial Hospital and Hagedorn Research Laboratory in 1981 to continue work on studies of the insulin gene region. In 1982, Owerbach and Nerup published an article in *Diabetes* that described the association of insulin gene polymorphism with diabetes mellitus [3]. The working hypothesis for this study was that polymorphism that gave rise to changes in the insulin molecule and thereby in the function of the insulin could be of pathogenetic significance for non-insulin-requiring diabetes. The article describes a positive association observed in a comparison of 47 insulin-independent diabetes patients and 93 control individuals. The authors had chosen a control group that consisted of two separate groups, namely 37 individuals with IDDM and 56 blood donors. In reality, the significant observation in the study is due to a difference between the NIDDM and IDDM groups, whereas there was no significant difference between the NIDDM and blood donor groups or the IDDM and blood donor groups. Owerbach and Nerup concluded that an increased occurrence of the 'u allele' in NIDDM patients was probably the true observation. This was supported by unpublished observations from the group that showed a correlation between the u allele and glycaemic control assessed by HbA_{1c}. This does not appear from the abstract of the article, and even the authors themselves play down their observation, but it is a fact that this work is the first to show a link between insulin gene polymorphism and T1D. This is an observation that is normally ascribed to Graeme Bell's work from 1984.

The significance of non-classic HLA genes in the HLA region

The 1980s saw the appearance of a long series of publications on HLA and insulin gene polymorphism in relation to diabetes. The HLA and insulin gene regions were still the only established genetic loci of importance for type 1 diabetes, when after a research stay in California the present writer came to Steno Memorial Hospital in 1988. In the same year, the Danish group with Mogens Thomsen as first author had published a work that showed it to be probable that the so-called HLA class III region also contained T1D risk genes [4]. The work focused on complement genes, but as the strong linkage disequilibrium in the region was now known, the authors pointed out that other genes in this region could also be important. The concurrent mapping of the region had shown that the genes for the tumor-necrosis factor (TNF) alpha and beta were also localized to this region. This, together with the pathogenetic model for the development of type 1 diabetes, which had been developed at this time at Steno Memorial Hospital and Hagedorn Research Laboratory, meant that Nerup's group had begun to focus on immune response genes such as TNF, interleukin-1 (IL-1) and interferon (IFN) gamma as possible candidate genes for T1D. The present writer started as specialist registrar in October 1988. From the very first day I had the opportunity of working in the laboratory.

The beginning of the era of 'functional genomics'

During my study residence in California, I had worked with various molecular biological techniques, for example mutation scanning and genotyping. It was natural to use these methods in studies of T1D. In a series of elegant studies, Jens Mølvig had shown that there were inter-individual differences in stimulated monocyte production of cytokines, among both healthy persons and T1D patients. We therefore chose to test whether these differences were conditioned by variations (polymorphism) in the genes that coded for these cytokines. Molecular genetic studies were a great challenge at this time. Sequences were known for only a limited number of genes, and in almost all cases only that part of the DNA was known that was transcribed. This made it difficult to localize the placing of polymorphism and thereby reduced the possibility of assessing causality. In a series of studies from 1990 to 1993, we showed that for both TNF and IL-1 beta there were gene polymorphisms that correlated with the amount of secreted protein [5-7]. For both TNF and IL-1 beta, we were able to show that this was an allele dose effect, so that persons who were homozygotic (i.e. were carriers of two copies of the variant) for the polymorphisms identified produced most protein. An interesting and still unexplained observation was that diabetes patients always had higher levels than healthy individuals with the same TNF and IL-1 genotype. These studies were perhaps the first, and were at any rate among the earliest, functional genetic studies in the field of diabetes. The findings were soon confirmed by other groups, and today the works are among the most cited of those that have been published from Steno Diabetes Center in the last 15 years.

Moreover, our own studies showed that the classic T1D-disposed HLA DR3 and DR4 haplotypes were identical at the TNF locus: both haplotypes coded for high TNF production. The heterozygotic form DR3/DR4, which is linked with the greatest risk of T1D, was thus associated with particularly high TNF production – an observation that made good pathogenetic sense [7].

Our own and others' subsequent studies showed that a combination of variations (haplotypes) in the individual gene regions correlated even better with the capacity for cytokine production.

Furthermore, candidate gene studies gave us indications that there might be differences in genetic risk profile in respect of non-HLA genes among familial and sporadic T1D patients [8]. In 6-8 % of cases, newly diagnosed patients have a first-degree relative with T1D, but after 30 years of diabetes the figure is as high as 25-30 % [9]. This has not been addressed in subsequent studies, but is of great importance for the interpretation of family-based versus case-control studies.

The hunt for non-HLA genes

It became clear at an early stage that intelligent pathogenesis model-based guesses might perhaps lead us to new T1D genes, but that large – very large – family studies would be necessary to find such non-HLA genes of relevance for the development of T1D.

The first family-based linkage studies were published from England, France and the USA. They were relatively small and the patient and control materials examined were of mixed ethnic background. Except for the HLA region, which all studies re-found, there was *no consistency in the findings among the studies.* Therefore, in 1996, we started an EU-financed joint project with groups in Norway, Sweden, France, Spain and Greece with a view to collecting and genotyping a very large number of Scandinavian families, which could only be regarded as considerably more genetically homogeneous than the previously investigated population groups. The expectation was that the use of a genetically homogeneous population would increase the strength of the study. But – neither did we find non-HLA loci that were the same as in previous publications [10].

When we reviewed the findings in the literature and the entire situation, it became clear to us that the existing methods for analyzing this type of data were not optimal. The methods were not suited for identifying genes with a small effect or with an effect that was present only in interaction with other genes. Colleagues in England and the USA had reached the same conclusion. It was a crisis! Also those holding the purse strings began to show signs of concern. Everybody was thinking about the question: what do we do now? The general conclusion was that as the effect of the single non-HLA gene was probably very small, the family materials had to be made larger. For hours and days on end, Nerup and I discussed the problem and on the basis of our pathogenesis model and our islet studies reached the conclusion that while the effect of a non-HLA gene in itself was small – i.e. only a fraction of the HLA effect, which could alone be calculated to about 50 % of the total effect – it was sufficiently large in interaction with other non-HLA genes. But how could we study this? As so often before, we found ideas outside the traditional diabetes research environment.

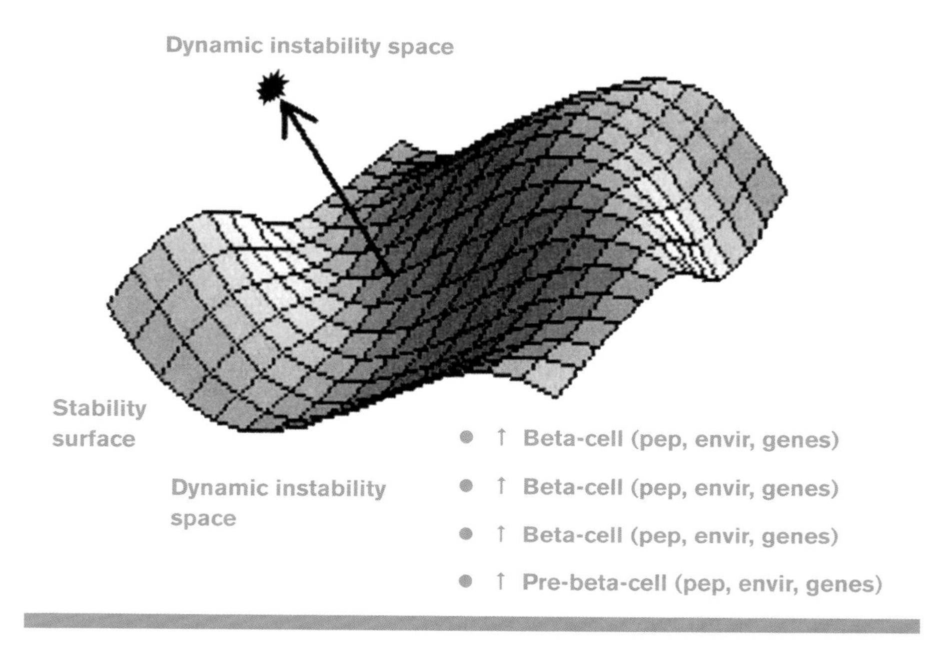

The beta-cell in a state of dynamic stability separated by a virtual surface from a state of dynamic instability. The pre-beta-cell is resistant to the toxic effect of cytokines and chemical toxins such as streptozotocin, and is at a good distance from the virtual surface. Through its final maturation, the resistance to cytokines and toxins is lost via changes in the cell's protein expression pattern (PEP). If the maturation of the beta-cell takes place under unfavourable conditions, e.g. in utero *in a pregnant rat on a reduced protein diet, receptivity to the toxic effects of cytokines and toxins is increased through further changes in PEP, and the beta-cell comes closer to the stability surface. If such PEP changes occur in beta-cells from genetically disposed individuals, the beta-cell moves dangerously close to the surface and can easily be pushed from a state of dynamic stability to a state dominated by dynamic instability and beta-cell death. (Commentaries on Perspectives in Diabetes, vol. 1, 1988-92. American Diabetes Association).*

Mathematics brought in to help

At the end of the 1990s, two things happened that would have great importance for our continued work on genetics and the pathogenesis approach in connection with T1D. At a meeting, Allan E Karlsen and I heard a presentation by representatives from the IT firm NeuroTech A/S. They described a study that on the basis of a large number of variables could predict what customers could be expected to renew their mobile phone subscription after the expiry of the discount period and what customers would switch to a new company in order to obtain yet another discount period from a new supplier. Their methods were based on decision tree algorithms and neural networks, i.e. *data mining*, and made us wonder whether such methods might also be used to analyze genetic data. This was the start of a collaboration over many years, in which we have developed, tested and published a number of new algorithms for the analysis of large amounts of genotyping data, and have been the first to show that multiple gene-gene interactions have an effect on the genetic disposition for T1D [11].

More or less at the same time, Per Bak, who was professor of theoretical physics at the Niels Bohr Institute, turned up at Nerup's office. He had read one of our articles and thought that we "*had entirely misunderstood our experimental observations from the laboratory trials that tested this model. The model can be fully described and understood in mathematical language*".

It took a number of long meetings before we began to be able to understand each other. Per Bak's intellect was both imaginative and effervescent, but at the same time analytic and stringent. In the eyes of the theoretical physicist, we were probably more imaginative and effervescent than stringent. But the 'chemistry' between us was good all the time, and together with Per Bak and one of his PhD students, Birgitte Freiesleben de Blasio, we developed in a very inspiring collaboration a mathematical model that described the earliest pathogenetic processes in T1D on the basis of our pathogenesis model. Although complicated mathematical formulas were required to describe these processes, the conclusion was surprisingly simple: namely that the start of the disease process is due to the fact that cytokines and/or environmental factors induce a collective, dynamic instability in the beta-cell. That one single triggering factor should be responsible is improbable. In its furthest consequence, this means that the beta-cells in an individual with considerable genetic risk for T1D will be situated as close to the interphase between dynamic stability and instability that even minor, non-specific – and perhaps even stochastic (random) – events are able to push the beta-cell from the stability phase over into the instability phase towards destruction and thereby diabetes.

The collaboration resulted in a major article in *Diabetes* in 1999 [12], which was clearly among the very best works from the group over the years – but also clearly one of the least frequently cited!

Both these cooperative projects convinced us that traditional reductionist ways of thinking and experiments were unlikely to lead us to the full understanding of the genetics and pathogenesis in T1D. It was thus inspired by physicists and mathematicians to 'think out of the box' that Nerup and I took the initiative for the already mentioned Skaw meeting.

Type 1 Diabetes Genetics Consortium – the future

Whether it was the long hikes across the dunes at Råbjerg Mile, the many hours in comfortable armchairs in the lounge or Jürg Ott's Scott Joplin music played on Hotel Kokholm's piano that finally produced a result must remain unsaid. At The Skaw meeting, it proved possible to agree on a declaration on cooperation regarding data, results and analyses. The first ideas concerning the financing of such activities were aired. This meeting was in reality the basis for the establishment of Type 1 Diabetes Genetics Consortium, T1DGC, a couple of years later. Already in November 2000, six months after Skaw, a broader circle of type 1 diabetes genetic researchers met in Rockville, Maryland, USA, with representatives from the National Institutes of Health (NIH) and the Juvenile Diabetes Research Foundation (JDRF) to discuss the possibilities for the structure of such an initiative. As a result of these meetings, the T1DGC was formed in September 2002 financed by NIDDK and JDRF [13]. Since the establishment of T1DGC, a large part of the genetic research has taken place under the auspices of this consortium. Huge new linkage analyses, whole genome association studies and candidate gene studies have been carried out [14]. The consortium is a unique model for how cooperation on data generation and analyses can strengthen the possibilities of isolating the genetic foundation for multifactorial disease, in this case type 1 diabetes.

In the current years, biomedical research is being driven forward by gene technology and powerful bioinformatics platforms with high capacities. At Steno Diabetes Center, we have in recent years focused on combining the accessible genetic data with other types of data, such as gene expression data and protein interaction data, so-called *systems biology* – an approach that will hopefully contribute to a more complete understanding of the aetiology and pathogenesis of T1D [15, 16]. In the midst of this profusion of huge studies and multidisciplinary joint projects generating mega amounts of data that are analysed in super-complex systems, we in our group are well aware how vital it is to maintain a research focus over time – often over a long period of time – and perhaps most importantly that there is space for an individual researcher to think a thought that no one has previously thought.

At the end of the 17th century, more or less at the same time as de Graaf, Harvey, Redi and Swammerdam, Niels Steensen formulated the theory that all female beings, including women, produced eggs, the first significant foundation for our understanding of *heredity* [17]. A good 325 years later, we at Steno Diabetes Center, in collaboration with colleagues from all around the world and with a common point of departure in ideas and findings from the early 1970s, are closer than ever before to identifying the genetic basis for type 1 diabetes.

REFERENCES

1. *Nerup J, Platz P, Andersen OO, Christy M, Lyngsøe J, Poulsen JE, Ryder LP, Staub-Nielsen L, Thomsen M, Svejgaard A. HL-A antigens and diabetes mellitus. Lancet 1974;ii:864-6*
2. *Thomsen M, Platz P, Andersen OO, Christy M, Lyngsøe J, Nerup J, Rasmussen K, Ryder LP, Nielsen LS, Svejgaard A. MLC typing in juvenile diabetes mellitus and idiopathic Addison's disease. Transplant Rev 1975;22:125-47*
3. *Owerbach D, Nerup J. Restriction fragment length polymorphism of the insulin gene in diabetes mellitus. Diabetes 1982;31:275-7*
4. *Thomsen M, Mølvig J, Zerbib A, de Preval C, Abbal M, Dugoujon JM, Ohayon E, Svejgaard A, Cambon-Thomsen A, Nerup J. The susceptibility to insulin-dependent diabetes mellitus is associated with C4 allotypes independently of the association with HLA-DQ alleles in HLA-DR3,4 heterozygotes. Immunogenetics 1988;28:320-7*
5. *Pociot F, Mølvig J, Wogensen L, Worsaae H, Dalbøge H, Baek L, Nerup J. A tumour necrosis factor beta gene polymorphism in relation to monokine secretion and insulin-dependent diabetes mellitus. Scand J Immunol 1991;33:37-49*
6. *Pociot F, Mølvig J, Wogensen L, Worsaae H, Nerup J. A TaqI polymorphism in the human interleukin-1ß (IL-1ß) gene correlates with IL-1ß secretion in vitro. Eur J Clin Invest 1992;22:396-402*
7. *Pociot F, Briant L, Jongeneel CV, Worsaae H, Mølvig J, Abbal M, Thomsen M, Nerup J, Cambon-Thomsen A. Association of tumor necrosis factor (TNF) and class II MHC alleles with the secretion of TNFa and TNFß by human mononuclear cells: A possible link to insulin-dependent diabetes mellitus. Eur J Immunol 1993;23:224-31*
8. *Pociot F, Rønningen KS, Bergholdt R, Lorenzen T, Johannesen J, Ye K, Dinarello CA, Nerup J, and the Danish Study Group of Diabetes in Childhood. Genetic susceptibility markers in Danish patients with type 1 diabetes – evidence for polygenecity in man. Autoimmunity 1994;19:169-78*

9. *Lorenzen T, Pociot F, Hougaard P, Nerup J. Long-term risk of IDDM in first-degree relatives of patients with IDDM. Diabetologia 1994;37:321-27.*
10. *Nerup J, Pociot F. European Consortium for IDDM genome Studies. A genome-wide scan for type 1 diabetes susceptibility genes in Scandinavian families. Identification of new loci with evidence of interaction. Am J Hum Genet 2001;69:1301-13*
11. *Pociot F, Karlsen AE, Petersen CB, Aalund M, Nerup J. Novel analytical methods applied to type 1 diabetes genome scan data. Am J Hum Genet 2004;74:647-60*
12. *Freiesleben B, Bak P, Pociot F, Karlsen AE, Nerup J. Onset of IDDM: a dynamic instability. Diabetes 1999;48:1677-85*
13. *Pociot F. The relevance of international consortia in studies on the pathogenesis of type 1 diabetes. The role of ET1DGN. Diabetes Metab Res Rev 2006;22:238-40*
14. *Type 1 Diabetes Genetics Consortium (Concannon P, Erlich HA, Julier C, Morahan G, Nerup J, Pociot F, Todd JA, Rich S). Type 1 Diabetes: Evidence for susceptibility loci from four genome-wide scans in 1435 multiplex families. Diabetes 2005;54:2995-3001*
15. *Bergholdt B, Karlsen AE, Hagedorn PH, Aalund M, Nielsen JH, Kruhøffer M, Ørntoft T, Wang H, Wollheim CB, Nerup J, Pociot F. Transcriptional profiling of type 1 diabetes genes on chromosome 21 in a rat beta-cell line and human pancreatic islets. Genes Immun 2007;8:232-8*
16. *Lage K, Karlberg EO, Størling ZM, Ólason PÍ, Pedersen AG, Rigina O, Hinsby AM, Tümer ZT, Pociot F, Tommerup N, Moreau Y, Brunak S. A human phenome-interactome network of protein complexes in genetic disorders. Nat Biotechnol 2007;25:309-16*
17. *Cobb M. The egg and sperm race: The seventeenth century scientists who unravelled the secrets of life, sex and growth. London: Free, 2006*

TYPE 2 DIABETES: FROM PHENOTYPE TO GENOTYPE AND BACK AGAIN

OLUF BORBYE PEDERSEN

My subject is broad and deep, and in this experiment at casting light on the national contributions, I am neither objective, balanced nor exhaustive, but on the contrary, influenced by the eyes that see and saw the world of yesterday. My wish is that my retrospect and the free associations that this has given rise to may be experienced by the reader as an invitation to dialogue and self-reflection. Only sporadically, towards the end of this essay, are there thoughts about the currents that no one knows – the future.

Snapshot of a day in the greenhouse

A Wednesday morning in April 1974. A busy day. As registrar I was halfway through the rounds in Medical Department 3, Århus County Hospital – a department of internal medicine specialising in diabetes and metabolic diseases. Just as I was examining a patient who had been admitted the previous evening with newly diagnosed diabetes, my chief came into the 6-bed ward and asked whether I had time to come to his office that afternoon at 4.30 for a staff meeting for the research-interested doctors. And there we were then: Kaj Erik Wildenhof, Leif Mosekilde, Torsten Toftegaard Nielsen, Jens Peter Bagger, Henning Beck-Nielsen and I – seated around Schwartz Sørensen and his coffee table. Before our arrival, he had brewed coffee in his kitchenette and fetched a portion of our indispensable afternoon speed – *the cookies.*

For the next almost two hours, he filled the room with his extraordinarily comprehensive knowledge of biochemistry and metabolism. The atmosphere was charged; his ideas sparkled, moved in many directions – rarely in a direct line and as a rule without a restricting structure. They were like small and large explosions. The sparks caught, for we were curious and intellectually hungry. We listened. Sometimes in wonderment, admiration, enchantment. At other times we – like the Master himself – lost the thread.

Without wishing to retouch the past or give way to idealizing nostalgia, I have to say that on those afternoons once or twice a month when we were invited to participate in the scientific coffee club, we sat under a star. An authentic star that had one goal: to shine for others. It was only later that I heard of research chiefs that most of all made me think of the Dead Sea, who had apparently never grasped the rewards to be won from passing on what is given to us as a loan and to be shared with others.

From "it's just maturity onset diabetes" to receptor biology

Niels Schwartz Sørensen trained under Hans Christian Hagedorn at Steno Memorial Hospital and had defended his doctoral dissertation on liver phosphorylase at the University of Copenhagen in 1960. Shortly afterwards, he came to Århus where, in 1964, he was appointed consultant at the Department of Medicine, Århus County Hospital. Its neighbour, Århus Municipal Hospital, had a medical-endocrinological department that had been headed by Knud Lundbæk since 1935. It was by no means easy to do pioneering work in the shadow of Lundbæk's productive research environment, and almost 10 years would pass before the neighbouring department fully recognized that original metabolism research was taking place at the County Hospital. In particular, I think that it meant a lot that Hans Ørskov from the competing department early on became aware of the Schwartz Sørensen team's potential and provided discreet, but vital, support.

At the start of the 1970s, the large group of diabetes patients who did not require insulin treatment to survive attracted little attention from the majority of Danish doctors. Many probably regarded the condition as relatively innocuous and one of the inevitable and natural consequences of ageing. Schwartz Sørensen did not share that view. Through his comprehensive studies of the literature – also the epidemiological literature – and from what he saw with his own eyes in his daily clinical work, he questioned whether the disease was as benign as some people appeared to assume. He was impressed by Himsvorth's works from 1939, which showed that a large proportion – perhaps even the majority – of diabetes patients were characterized by a reduced insulin effect. Schwartz Sørensen's vision was that his research group should begin a systematic project to characterize insulin sensitivity at cell and whole body level in those who were obese and in diabetes patients who did not require insulin treatment.

On 1 May 1973, Henning and I began as registrars in the Department. A few days later, we were summoned to the chief's office. The atmosphere was electric. Schwartz Sørensen was excited and enthused. He had just returned from a congress, at which American research groups presented further experimental support for the existence of a receptor for insulin.

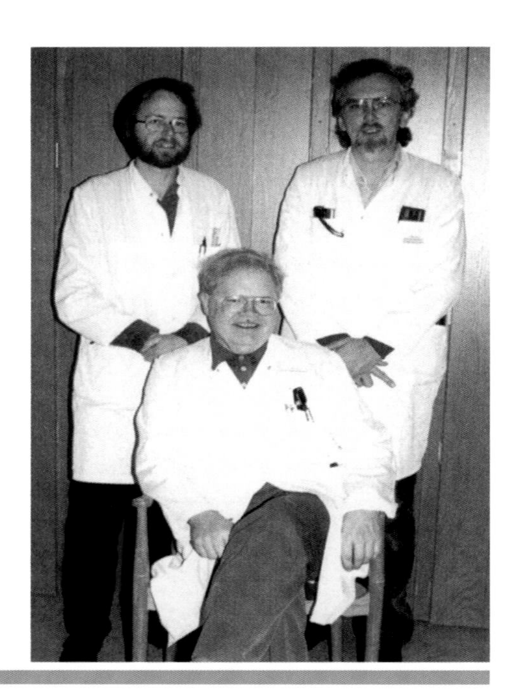

Oluf Pedersen (left) and Henning Beck-Nielsen behind the master Niels Schwartz Sørensen.

The first tender shoots of a breakthrough in the form of an incipient cellular-biological understanding of insulin's receptor-binding had come from Crofford's, Cuatrecasas' and Roth's laboratories in 1969–71. We couldn't help being infected by his contagious eagerness to pursue and expand the receptor finds on Danish soil and in a clinical context, and when we were asked whether on top of our work as registrars we were willing to devote a substantial part of our energy and free time to such a project, we promptly answered in the affirmative, even before the commitment and investment of time had been discussed with our families. Today, 34 years later in a Danish family of academics, it would scarcely be possible to take decision of such import with the same speed! For Henning and me, this became the beginning of a new way of life rather than of a new form of work. Although there was initially a natural competitiveness between us, we soon developed a collaboration in which we developed and integrated each other's strong sides. As a catalyst for the process, Schwartz Sørensen was unusual – not least because of his personal humility, and because he helped his young researchers to grow and mature both as human beings and as specialists by giving them space in the form of unreserved confidence and unlimited attention.

Open Danish doors

Perhaps, with the exception of the future, there is very little that comes by itself, and certainly not progress. This rephrasing of a saying by the well-known Danish lamp designer and thinker Poul Henningsen aptly described the state in which we found ourselves during the first six months in the research basement at Århus County Hospital. After many attempts and with guidance from American laboratories, we succeeded in isolating sufficiently pure suspensions of lymphocytes and later of the insulin-receptor enriched monocytes from peripheral blood. We thus had easily accessible cells, which we assumed at that time reflected the insulin-receptor in those of the body's cells that had far greater quantitative importance for carbohydrate and fat metabolism: namely, muscle, fat and liver cells. This was an assumption that Elisabeth Hjøllund in her later dissertation work showed did not hold under a number of biological conditions. It remained to procure 125-monoiodine insulin with sufficiently high specific activity to allow us to measure the specific receptor-binding with sufficient precision. Jens Højriis Nielsen from Hagedorn Research Laboratory, Jørgen Gliemann, Steen Gammeltoft and Ole Sonne from the Physiological Institute, University of Copenhagen, and not least the director of Novo's Research Institute, Lise Heding, gave us invaluable advice and materials. Even though the first radioactive cell markings were – not entirely without a health risk – captured with Geiger-Müller tubes, it took only 18 months before standardized and safe methods for measuring insulin-receptor binding had been established and validated in the research basement.

Developments gather speed

Together with Jørgen Gliemann, I developed methods for isolating viable human fat cells that I took in biopsies from the gluteal region of hundreds of volunteer patients and trial persons in order to illuminate new links between receptor-binding and the insulin's cellular effect of glucose transport, lipogenesis, lipid oxidation and antilipolysis at cell level. After my doctoral dissertation in 1983, Elisabeth Hjøllund expanded the comparative insulin-receptor studies, while Jens Friis Bak set up and applied methods for measuring insulin-receptor binding and receptor kinase activity in muscle biopsies from humans and compared receptor findings with the ability of insulin to stimulate glycogen synthesis. Bjørn Richelsen and later Steen Bønløkke Pedersen continued work on fat cell receptor biology for a number of hormones other than insulin and insulin-regulated cell signalling and metabolism. With independent measures, we had succeeded in developing *state of the art* technologies *in vitro* and *in vivo* for collecting valuable new knowledge on a number of pathophysiological and cellular-biological mechanisms, not least insulin resistance. The research basement buzzed with the activities of colourful personalities. There was light in the windows from early morning to late evening – sometimes right until the next morning when the 24-hour rhythms of metabolites and receptors were being studied, and family members came with picnic baskets in order to bring the necessary fuel to the over-zealous researchers. There were few compromises, standards were high and mediocrity had a hard time of it. The laboratory had been recognized and had acquired a reputation – and visiting researchers came to stay with us.

Meeting with international research

There is a great potential for development in the meeting with the other. A powerful poetic example is falling in love and its possible consequences. Those blazing fires that take hold out of which something new emerges, for those who are receptive, occur often – also in professional life. In the early phase of the Århus group's development, the meeting with Gerald Reaven from Stanford University was crucial. It was my experience that like other people with major gifts, he had learnt to compensate for an inborn urge towards narcissism and self-aggrandizement by developing his tolerance and insight and thereby finding room to give recognition to others. We were among those who benefited. C Ronald Kahn, from the National Institute of Health in Washington and later at the Joslin Diabetes Center, Harvard, saw in us a reflection of his aims and interests and thereby became a vital inspiration for our initiatives. When Henning and I had completed our specialist training, we both went to the USA to study, Henning to the University of California in San Diego and I to the Joslin Diabetes Center at Harvard. Our stays in the new growth zones undoubtedly helped us to avoid getting stuck in autodidacticism and, seen in a global perspective, provincialism. The research environment at Harvard was electric. New thinking was encouraged, there were many talented researchers, and nobody was allowed just to sit back and relax. Starting up in the laboratory was like a test of one's survival skills. Table space in the lab, equipment, chemicals, experimental animals – everything was up for competition. New personal qualities were stimulated and cultivated, and the insight from the many experiments was rewarding. I arrived at Joslin at the very time when the new signalling proteins were being cloned and described, and when the first glucose transport proteins had been identified. Furthermore, Barbara Kahn and Jeffrey Flier from Beth Israel Hospital invited me to work on wildly exciting studies of links between insulin-stimulated glucose transport activity and transport protein expression at protein and mRNA level. My family – and I with it – blossomed in this privileged enclave of the American way of life.

Time of crisis from 1988 to 1992

In 1988, I returned to Denmark. There was no lack of cautionary advice from colleagues at home and abroad. Some were of the opinion that the Copenhagen diabetes research environment was "over the hill", and one person jointly labelled the two Copenhagen diabetes hospitals and their owner as "a sunset enterprise". Nevertheless, I made the move to Copenhagen, to Steno Diabetes Center. But the first years were not the best. The big names were there: Deckert, Binder, Nerup and Parving. Different, of course. Some with the classical virtues as people and leaders. Others in manifesting their life expression – entirely themselves. All four colleagues were helpful. Their research was well-established and almost exclusively rooted in type 1 diabetes. Numerous important results had long been published and had made an international impact. The environment was rich in tradition with stimulating literature evenings and a well equipped laboratory at Hagedorn, but it was all a touch old-fashioned and stuffy. I was astonished when almost as an echo I heard that type 2 diabetes was probably not actually diabetes! Fogginess – what in the world had I got myself into? As a consequence of this and to create for myself the necessary free space for clarifying what my possible future in Copenhagen might be, I at times in the first years chose quiet retreats at the manor houses of Fuglsang and Vedbygaard. Even though Schwartz Sørensen wanted me back in his chair, in the end I decided to stay at Steno. After a couple of years, I succeeded in getting molecular biological laboratory facilities at Hagedorn and later in Bagsværd thanks to generosity at Novo Nordisk's headquarters. While waiting, in a flexible and fruitful cooperation with Per Heden Andersen, Steen Lund and Ole Schmitz, we implemented at the Århus laboratory the molecular biological methods I had learnt at Harvard, and under the guidance of Geoffrey Holman from Bath, we incorporated in our repertoire techniques for studies of the translocation of glucose transport proteins in muscle tissue.

Two parallel tracks from 1991: intervention studies of gene variants in metabolic diseases

Out of the quietness and the manor house Fuglsang's open meadows by Guldborg Sound and through inspiration from a number of the guests at the retreat (thoughtful scientists and artists) came two ideas and, at the same time and just as importantly, the *courage* to pursue them. One idea was to initiate a clinical trial in order to elucidate whether at all it was appropriate and justified in the long term to treat type 2 diabetes patients multifactorially. No one knew, and in this field many clinicians appeared to entertain a certain defeatism, indeed perhaps nihilism. In January 1991, I presented to my consultant colleagues at Steno my protocol for the project I later named

"The Steno 2 Study". The spontaneous support failed to materialize, and it was not until January 1993 that the trial proper could begin. And adverse winds continued to blow. Not least, the reaction from Steno's international Peer Review Board was totally devoid of constructive support. With a joy that had *no* foundation and an unaltered belief in the rightness of the research idea, the work continued for the life of the project. In July 1995, four and a half years after the presentation of the project, I invited Hans-Henrik Parving to join the steering group for "Steno 2". With his enthusiasm, he was a great asset. Pernille Vedel wrote her Ph.D. thesis on the project's early phase, and with insight and empathy, Peter Gæde went on to conduct the intervention together with the multidisciplinary team.

The main findings were published in *The Lancet* and *The New England Journal of Medicine*, and in 2007, we have concluded the 13-year survey, which shows that intensive multifactorial intervention in respect of the known risk markers cuts mortality and the occurrence of disease in small and large blood vessels by half. At the same time, the health-economic analyses show that the cost-effectiveness is all right. A ray of sunshine through the fog.

The other research idea from 1991 couldn't be realized fast enough. The idea was to combine molecular genetics, gene expression, protein chemistry and physiological studies to cast light on the importance of possible gene variants for metabolic phenotypes. Once again it was a little like running a marathon on loose dry sand. Without the unparalleled generosity – in the form of a personal gift – of the Kann Rasmussen family, a central branch of which had acquired and settled in my childhood home, we would probably never have attained an international flying altitude. The seven-figure donations were invested in advanced gene technology apparatus.

The first harvest among monogenic forms of metabolic disease

Two brothers of 15 and 8 years of age, they had been referred to Steno from a different part of the country because of hyperinsulinaemia (45-90 times above the highest normal value). One of them had diabetes, the other reduced glucose tolerance. Henrik Vestergård described in detail the pathophysiology behind their severe insulin resistance and the disturbances in their sugar metabolism. With help from the Pierre De Meyts group at Hagedorn, the molecular pathogenesis was characterized: both had two mutations in the gene that codes for the insulin-receptor. One mutation was inherited from a healthy mother; the other from a healthy father. But together the two mutations in the children resulted in a loss of virtually 100 % of normal insulin signalling and effect. A molecular genetic triumph, but for the patients and us a deep disappointment because we are still unable to translate this precise

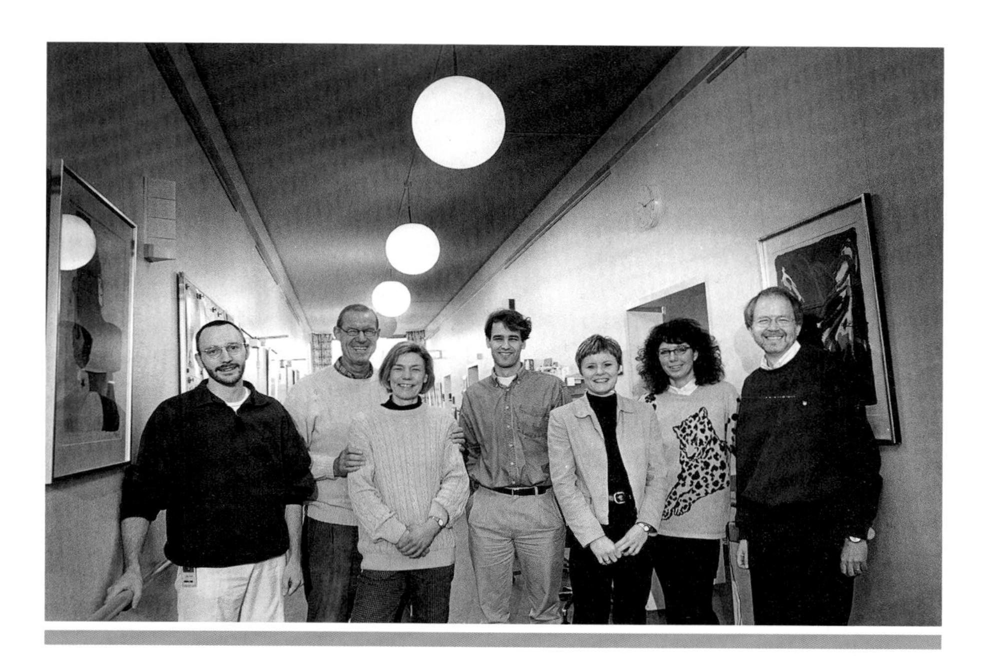

The assistants at the birth of the Steno 2 Study, 1999.
From the left: Jacob Obel, Hans-Henrik Parving, Bente Blaaholm Nielsen. Peter Gæde, Susanne Kohlwes, Maiken Beck and Oluf Pedersen.

pathogenetic understanding into compensatory, targeted treatment. I draw attention to this example as an illustration of the impressive breakthroughs there have been in the course of just a few years in our understanding of the causes of many monogenic diseases. But at the same time, there is a long way to go for the majority of these genetically speaking relatively easily accessible diseases before our molecular insight can benefit the patients. This is a lesson in humility in the face of the extent of the challenges and the unchanged burdens to be borne by the patients.

A far brighter picture emerges in respect of the autosomal and monogenic form of diabetes with onset before the age of 25, which is in English called *Maturity Onset Diabetes of the Young (MODY)*. MODY is estimated to constitute 1-2 % of all diabetes disorders. We were quick off the mark and were included in the international consortium that Graeme Bell in Chicago headed, and which in 1995 led to the publication in *Nature* of the first diabetes gene that explained the most frequent form of MODY, and which has now been given the designation MODY3. It can be caused by many different mutations in the gene that codes for the transcription factor, hepatic nuclear factor 1 alfa. Since then, other MODY genes (6 in all) have been found and described, which together explain just over half of all MODY cases. Besides a large amount of new knowledge on the biology of the insulin-producing beta-cells, this has resulted in what is concretely formulated in the title of this essay: *from phenotype to genotype and back again*. The mildest form, MODY2, is due to mutations in the gene for glucokinase. As a rule, the patients need no pharmacological treatment and rarely develop complications. The opposite is the case for MODY3. Many patients experience a relatively aggressive course, at least at the same level as for classical type 1 diabetes. The surprising thing is, however, that the patients can often benefit from treatment with sulfonylurea tablets instead of insulin. In other words, one of the first real successes with genotype-based pharmacological treatment. In an exemplary collaboration with Jørn Nerup, Flemming Pociot, Peter Damm and their groups, we have shown that not an insignificant number of MODY patients are concealed (and are incorrectly treated) among type 1 diabetes patients and patients with gestational diabetes. Torben Hansen, a talented and committed scientist and my partner in the research group for 10 years, has been the architect and driving force behind the work to achieve an understanding of the causes of the monogenic metabolic diseases. Thanks to his efforts, Steno has become a national centre for the diagnosis of these diseases.

Molecular genetic studies of polygenic metabolic diseases: no longer on all fours at last

In Denmark, there is a tradition for research into the hereditary factors behind the frequent forms of diabetes and obesity. Pioneering studies in diabetes were published by Hauge and Harvald and their group in the 1960s, and in the 1980s, Thorkild Sørensen and his team published their watershed studies of hereditability of obesity. More recently, the research tradition has been continued in a number of convincing twin studies by Henning Beck-Nielsen, Allan Vaag and Pernille Poulsen and their groups. As a simplified conclusion to the many contributions, it would seem to be a matter of a polygenic inheritance and heritabilities of 30-70 %. But from this point and until the first underwater currents in the form of specific disease genes linked to the frequent forms of type 2 diabetes and obesity could be identified would prove to be an unexpectedly long and demanding odyssey. In the beginning of the 1990s, we chose the pathophysiological approach to genome research. For instance, we qualified the genes on which we performed mutation analyses on the basis of results from published knockout experiments in mouse models. Often they were further qualified by information from our own or other researchers' studies of whether the gene was situated in an area of the genome for which a linkage disequilibrium had been demonstrated. Gradually, our patient materials became larger, which gave more statistical power in association studies and a higher degree of purity, i.e. made it possible for some of the clinical and thereby probably the hereditary heterogenicity to be eliminated. Crucial and extremely fruitful cooperation was established with Torben Jørgensen, Knut Borch-Johnsen, Torsten Lauritzen, Hans Ibsen, Thorkild Sørensen, Cramer Christensen and Ivan Brandslund as well as several others, which made it possible to perform genetic studies on more than 20,000 well-characterized study participants. In the years that have passed, there have been found a number of genes that are pathogenic in all investigated ethnic groups for type 2 diabetes or obesity, and about which there is agreement among international researchers. To these can be added a number of others that are being validated, and which may be pathogenic in some ethnic groups. On the basis of the publication of the first decodings of the human genome and the publication of HaPMap, which is a survey of frequent variants in the genome and their locus representativity, chips bearing up to 1 million genome markers have been developed. These advances in knowledge and technology have made it possible to carry out so-called whole genome association studies. Hereby more replicated gene variants have been identified, which contribute to explaining the pathogenesis of both type 2 diabetes and obesity. Yes, we have become sufficiently sure on our feet to be able to walk unaided – and there is much that looks extremely promising.

And what then?

Even though in genome research we are now able to stand upright and move relatively quickly, there still remain many challenges to be met before we have an overview of how many genes are in reality involved in the metabolic diseases, and how they interact mutually and with the innumerable known and unknown environmental and behavioural factors. And what about epigenetics and the importance of effects in the womb for health and disease, questions pursued with such focus by Allan Vaag and his group? There is undoubtedly a need both to puncture and let go of outdated ideas, to develop new paradigms for normality and illness and not least to validate and use higher order mathematics and *in vivo* imaging technologies for "traffic analyses" of the multiple genetic and non-genetic variables that enter into the equations. But already now on the horizon, we can glimpse the contours of pictures that suggest what the new knowledge concerning polygenic disease can be used for. The first thing that many people can see is genotype-based treatment and prevention of disease, and this applies for drugs and behaviour such as exercise and nutrition. The second thing may prove to be that genome markers, together with gender, age, anthropometric measurements and serum biomarkers will enter into algorithms for effective prophylaxis.

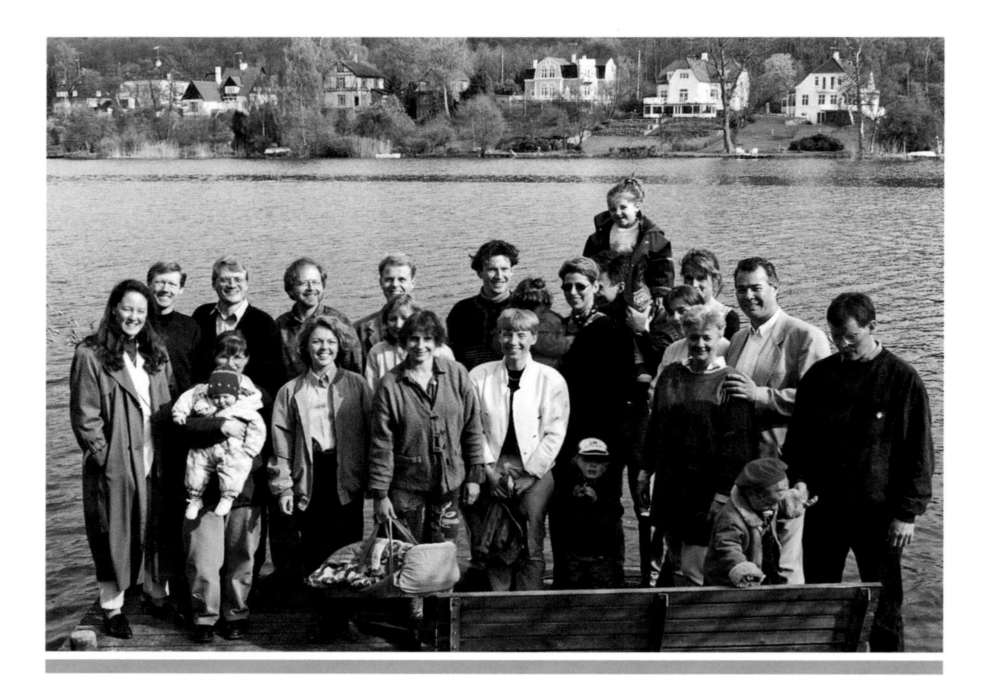

The author's vigorous research team in spring sunshine in 1995.

It is a lifestyle

Globalization has long since made its entry into Danish biomedical research. Larger research units with correspondingly heavy budgets and many alliances are a reality. For example, my research group has over the past 14 years largely been financed by 7 EU grants and has thereby been allied with more than 80 different European research groups.

Much has changed, but the ingredients that make things flower in research greenhouses that are characterized by both "bottom-up" and "top-down" initiatives seem to be the same as they were in the 1970s in Århus. Self-motivation must be stressed. In the "statutes" of my research group his is underlined as a reformulation of a Kennedy statement: "*Don't ask what your work community can do for you, but what you can do for your professional community and yourself*". Something else we give priority to is the formalized weekly meetings. For the individual staff member, there is the "11 minutes with the boss" and for the group as a whole, there is the 2-hour data- and journal-club in which youthful intellectual and creative cheekiness is confronted with the wisdom of the more experienced.

Courage, humour, endurance, curiosity, the fizzing of endorphins in enthusiasm over an idea or an insight, listening quietly, an abundance of appreciative attention from chief to staff and vice-versa, and encouragement for *daily* reading of idea-developing, original and survey articles in order to make it to the soloist class on one's scientific instrument, and not to forget flair for timing and speed in respect of data analysis and publication.

Translation into policy of important research results

Knowledge is perhaps one of our strongest tools in the struggle for survival. But in basic research and in applied research – not least in the fields of biotechnological and molecular genetic development – we have to deal with really complex tasks, and the research results may be difficult to communicate in an easily accessible syntax. Innovations are therefore perceived by some as a threat rather than as a message of freedom and a possibility of life with a greater potential and less suffering. It therefore seems to be vitally important that there should be voices that rise above the superficial everyday presentation of specialist knowledge by the media, and which *in public* insist on a rational and scientifically founded debate in which objective cognition is central. It is not enough to seek to achieve the highest possible scientific "*impact factor*". The corresponding "*impact factor*" for the resulting political consequences should be made far more attractive. As scientists it must be our responsibility to present new balanced results in a form that is accessible to politicians and therefore to their voters. If as communicating scientists we do not deliver the scientifically founded core in the health policy argumentation, one scarcely needs to be a dyed-in-the-wool pessimist to be able to foresee the absence of political initiatives that could prevent a situation in which in a few years' time more than three-quarters of all diseases will be due to lifestyle and modern community causes. The molecular genetic research into widespread diseases will undoubtedly help to explain the mismatch that exists between our only 60-year-old, sedentary, fat-saturated society and our genetic make-up, which millions of years of evolution have trimmed in order to secure an active life under quite different conditions. Will we be ready to act when perhaps in the relatively near future there is sufficient evidence on the table from international research into the interaction between genome and behaviour? Will we be able to persuade the governing minister of health of the benefits of *offering* the individual citizen a bio-marker profile to strengthen his or her motivation for lifelong health behaviour? A message of freedom? Or will it be a completely different ball game at that time?

GROWTH HORMONE AND DIABETIC ANGIOPATHY

HANS ØRSKOV

History and background

Once upon a time, it was in 1969, on a Thursday of course, or rather as the culmination of a series of Thursday rendezvous, we had gained sufficient courage and confidence (evidence) so we felt ready to propose. We proposed the "growth hormone hypothesis" [1] postulating that the diabetic growth hormone hypersecretion is a causal factor in the origin and development of diabetic angiopathy.

Knud Lundbæk became professor of internal medicine of 1953, Aarhus University, and founded a remarkable research unit. His cardinal interest was diabetic angiopathy, a concept he had defined himself [2, 3]. His perspicacity and skills as supervisor at-

THE LANCET, JULY 18, 1970

Hypothesis

DIABETES, DIABETIC ANGIOPATHY, AND GROWTH HORMONE

K. LUNDBÆK, N. JUEL CHRISTENSEN, VIGGO A. JENSEN, K. JOHANSEN, T. STEEN OLSEN, Å. PRANGE HANSEN, H. ØRSKOV, R. ØSTERBY

Second Clinic of Internal Medicine, Department of Ophthalmology, and Institute of Pathology, Aarhus University School of Medicine, Kommunehospitalet, Aarhus, Denmark

Summary Raised plasma-growth-hormone (G.H.) levels in juvenile diabetes, the persistence of abnormal G.H. response to exercise even in well-controlled diabetics, the inhibitory effect of hypophysectomy on the progression of diabetic retinopathy and the normalisation of skin capillary fragility after this operation all point to a role for G.H. hypersecretion in the development of diabetic angiopathy.

The Lancet article in which the growth hormone hypothesis was proposed

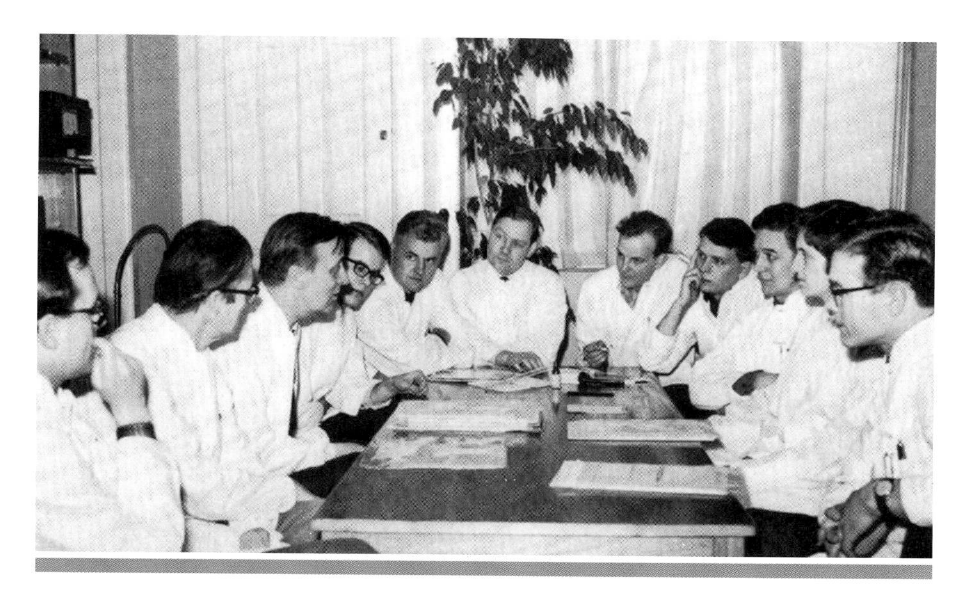

A Thursday conference, 1965: the guru and his disciples. From the left: Klaus Johansen, Sigurd Eskjær Jensen, Knud Lundbæk, Carl Erik Mogensen, Vagn Drewes, Hans Yde, Hans Ørskov, Niels Juel Christensen, Gunnar Gregersen, Ruth Østerby and Hans Agerbæk.

tracted immediately a series of hopeful students and young doctors. The second litter is seen in the photo taken in 1965 at a Thursday conference. He introduced these conferences, when he became professor, with the aim to accustom his pupils to present and discuss their recent results, to set these in perspective in relation to international and their colleagues' research and to learn to give and tolerate severe criticism. In this way, every Thursday continues to serve more than fifty years later.

An observer of the photo is in no doubt at whom the attention – no, fascination – is centered. And a presentation could be quite a nervous ordeal the first time; a few participants had to be resuscitated with a generous measure of Scotch before they could take up the thread.

Lundbæk was admired and feared by his medical students. At the final examination in internal medicine, he asked you to draw a card from a large box with 200 topics. My best friend in 1959 took "painful shoulders" – and we knew he was doomed. Lundbæk's favourite torture was partial rupture of the supraspinator muscle, and he asked: *"Which profession do you believe is particularly bothered?"* My friend closely observed his carotic arteries and his sphinx-like face, while he answered: *"Ceiling painters"* –

and instantly added: "*When they dip their brush*". I believe, he was the only student, who ever scored a decent mark in this topic.

In the sixties, there was already a long line of evidence connecting growth hormone to diabetes, or rather to insulin sensitivity, the most impressive being Rabinowitz and Zierler's famous experiments from 1963 with intraarterial infusions of growth hormone in the resting human forearm, demonstrating an immediate suppression of muscle glucose uptake and an approximately two hours delayed stimulation of lipolysis. Before that, convincing animal research had shown that long-term growth hormone administration induced permanent diabetes in dogs.

But to our knowledge, nobody had suggested a direct relationship between growth hormone and late diabetic cardiovascular manifestations. It is true that diabetes patients with proliferative retinopathy in especially Stockholm and London had been treated with pituitary ablation by hypophysectomy or implantation of radioactive yttrium. It must be considered that at that time, before the era of laser treatment, no therapies were available to delay or prevent blindness in patients with proliferative retinopathy. These experiments had received support to continue by Jakob Poulsen's description in 1953 of a patient whose severe retinopathy vanished after she postdelivery suffered panhypopituitarism through a Sheehan's syndrome [4]. Neither the Stockholm nor London studies were clinical controlled placebo experiments.

Lundbæk felt rightly that we should get nowhere until we mastered techniques for measurement of insulin and growth hormone. So a doctor was sent to Hammersmith Hospital in 1960 to be taught hypophysectomy in rats and returned with a circular filter paper on which were drawn 3 equal segments, the purpose being to place the anaesthetized head in the centre and insert a guided canula along one segment line into the sella through an ear. This technique was unsuccessful in Århus. We found, however, that newborn rats were equally sensitive to the "sulphation factor" and readily took up radiolabelled sulphate in costal cartilage fragments.

This chemically uncharacterized sulphation factor had been found to mediate growth hormone's mitogenic (growth) effects. It was later termed "somatomedin C" and still later, after characterisation, IGF-I.

Hans Yde found with the modified bioassay that juvenile (type 1) diabetes patients had markedly reduced sulphation factor activity in plasma and that the reduction was strongly reversely related to the average blood glucose [5].

This was sceptically received by Lundbæk (who, I think, had already intuitively decided that high growth hormone levels, and therefore also those of its mediator's, obtained in diabetes patients). Retrospectively, it was the first indication of the negative IGF-I/growth hormone feedback.

Before that, Jens Lyngsøe had taken up the rat epididymis fat technique in order to measure serum insulin. Fragments of fat tissue were incubated with serum or insulin standards and an insulin-like activity (ILA) was determined by measuring the turnover of radioactive glucose. ILA consisted of a part that could be suppressed by addition of antiinsulin antiserum, and the great majority called Non Suppressible Insulin–Like Activity (NSILA), which later was identified as IGF-I plus IGF-II.

Years later, it occurred to us that Yde and Lyngsøe had been unaware that they measured with two very different bioassays practically the same substance, possibly even in the same serum samples.

In 1960, Yalow & Berson had invented the radioimmunoassay, and in 1962, Hales & Randle made an easier modification "the double antibody assay"; so the same year, Lundbæk despatched me to Cambrigde to learn the pitfalls. However, upon return I introduced another more robust modification: wick chromatography, that became used in our laboratory during 25 years for a large number of hormones [6].

Yde found that radioimmunoassayable serum growth hormone responded in a paradoxical way to glucose in type 1 diabetes patients, it was stimulated instead of being suppressed. This was in contrast to the icons Yalow & Berson, who had claimed that growth hormone was normal in diabetes patients in this situation, but they were nuclear scientists and had not distinguished between the fat type 2 and the lean type 1 diabetes.

Aage Prange Hansen and Klaus Johansen took up the challenge of Yalow and Berson's dogma and found that type 1 diabetes patients had highly increased and early response to stimuli and a 3 times higher average 24 hour serum level compared to controls, and most importantly that this hypersecretion was related to blood glucose status and could be *almost* normalized during exceptionally strict metabolic control [7, 8]. Previously, Lundbæk and coworkers had undertaken the first (and only) controlled clinical trial of the effect of hypophysectomy on proliferative retinopathy and found in a small number of patients that vision was marginally but significantly less reduced in the hypophysectomized group.

The growth hormone hypothesis

These two findings became the foundation of the hypothesis:

1) Type 1 diabetes patients had hypersecretion of growth hormone from the onset of diabetes and for the rest of their lives, and this abnormality was dependent on metabolic control.
2) The hypophysectomy study had indicated that this intervention delayed progress of the retinopathy in patients who had received replacement of pituitary hormones except growth hormone.

3) In addition, Niels Juel Christensen had in 1968 published that the increased fragility of skin capillaries in type 1 diabetes was normalized in the hypophysectomised patients.

The proposed theory received attention. Some colleagues were sceptical. For instance because we were unable to explain why obese type 2 diabetes patients develop angiopathy, despite the fact that their serum growth hormone was suppressed to similar low levels as found in obese non-diabetes patients. We countered that their growth hormone concentrations were at or below the sensitivity limit of immunoassay in those days, and that obese subjects must be ultrasensitive to growth hormone pointing out that obese children grow normally. Another difficult point was the question why patients with acromegaly did not have galloping retinopathy, we never found any deadly repartee for that, except that these patients had high serum IGF-I, while diabetes patients had low serum IGF-I.

In general, the reaction to our hypothesis was characterized by kind and cautious interest. Partly, I suppose because everybody those days was hoping for a possible breakthrough in unravelling the pathogenesis of and thereby putative tools to combat angiopathy. At that time, many diabetologists had a defeatistic view of the benefit of metabolic control. Others had on the contrary particularly appreciated the demonstrated tight inverse relationship between metabolic control and hypersomatropinaemia.

At any rate, a prolific series of studies was triggered and is still going on in our centre as well as elsewhere to refute or sustain the validity of the theory – and to attempt to exploit its possibilities in prophylaxis and therapy.

Those who were sceptic concerning the utility of metabolic control were impressed by the American Siperstein, who had postulated that the basal membrane of small vessels was already thickened at the onset of diabetes, and therefore a genetic manifestation, whose progress would be independent of the metabolic state. We believed his measurements had been imprecise, and Ruth Østerby undertook her pioneer morphometric study and showed that accurate estimates of the basal membrane width could be obtained in photomontages of 20.000 times enlarged glomeruli and that it was entirely normal at diabetes debut.

In our team, an interesting extension of the theory to include macroangiopathy was indicated by Thomas Ledet's studies of cultured aortic smooth muscle cells. He found that added growth hormone in physiological concentrations stimulated the outgrowth and so did addition of diabetic serum, an effect which disappeared, when incubation took place with addition of anti growth hormone antiserum [9].

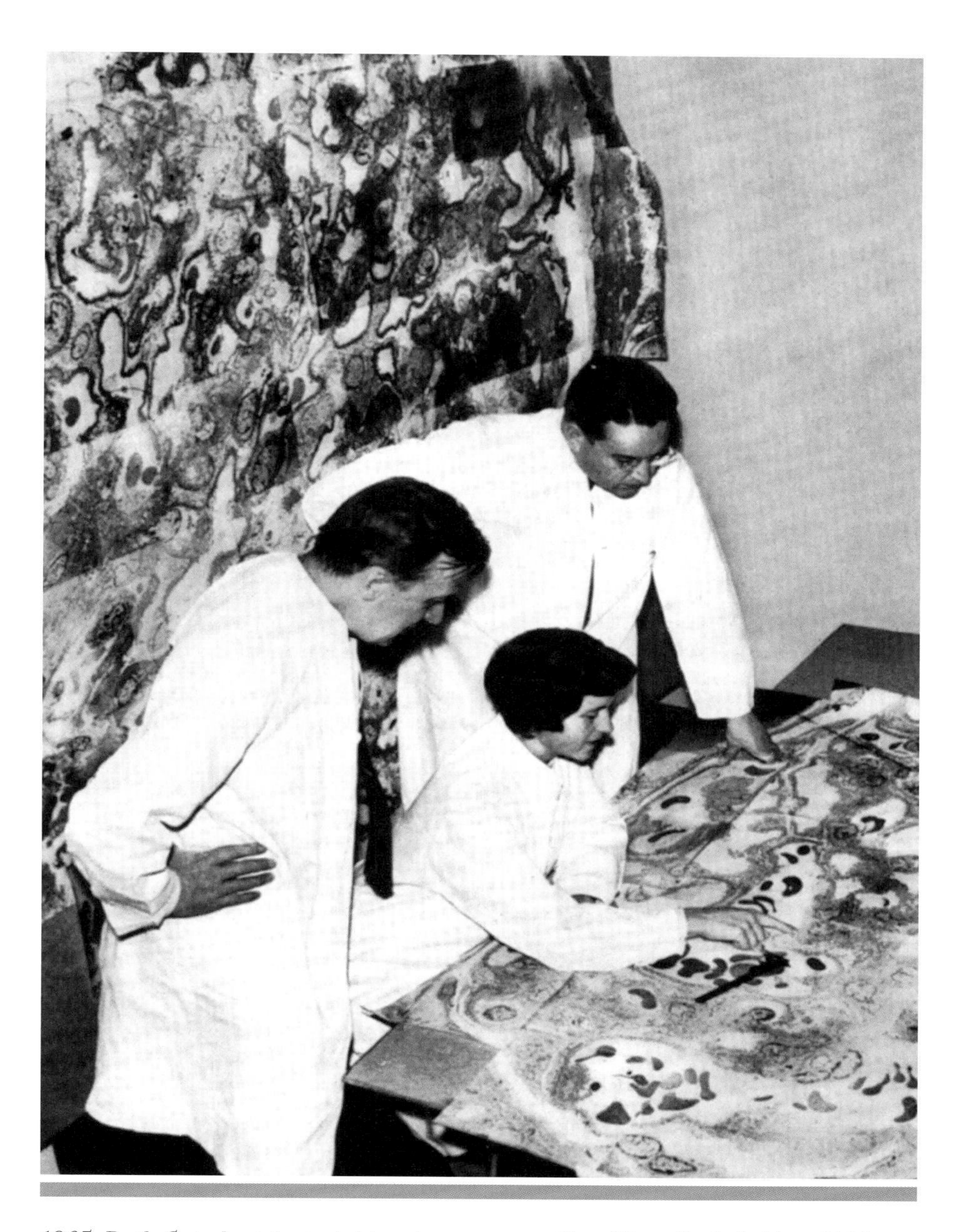

1965. Ruth Østerby tries to initiate her mentors, Knud Lundbæk (left) and T Steen Olsen, into the wondrous world of morphometrics. By her right hand can be seen the sliding gauge that she used to measure the basal membrane thickness on her 20,000 times magnified photomontages of electromicroscoped glomeruli.

The most striking support we received was Sharp and coworkers' follow-up study in 1987 of 100 patients after yttrium ablation of the pituitary in London in the sixties [10]. In brief, they found that retinal new vessel formation fell from 100 % (an inclusion criterion) over 3 years to less than 40 %, and after 10 years only 4 of the 42 survivors had any new vessel formation left. Vision was also better preserved than expected.

Surprisingly, they also found that the treated patients had lower cardiovascular mortality than expected from Torsten Deckert's pioneer study [11] of pituitary intact diabetic type 1 patients, again suggesting a possible role for growth hormone in diabetic large vessel disease. Curiously, this hitherto strongest supporter (Sharp) of our theory concluded in a review in 1993 after emphasising again the benefits of pituitary ablation and the diabetic growth hormone hypersecretion [12]: *"It is the opinion of the author that growth hormone does not play a direct role in the development of diabetic microvascular disease"!* (But he gave no persuasive evidence for his statement).

Further support was Merimee et al's demonstration that growth hormone deficient diabetic dwarfs did not develop retinopathy, even after a further 8 years follow-up [13, 14]. But it must be considered that their diabetes was mild.

Suppressing growth hormone hypersecretion

The observation that extremely strict metabolic control reduced plasma growth hormone was confirmed in several studies, but it soon became evident that complete long-term normalisation was unattainable. So we began to search amongst a great number of pharmaca, but found no expedient candidate.

Several pharmaceutical companies had become interested in our hypothesis. For example, Lundbæk and I were in 1971 invited to Hoffman la Roche's fortress and received a splendid reception. They had the idea that a solution might be development of an antagonist to the newly discovered growth hormone releasing hormone. We felt early that their plans had not approached action and that their prime object was to secure our signatures on an agreement, which would have bound us forever.

Two years later, Guillemin's group discovered the growth hormone release inhibitor, SRIF or somatostatin [15], and the Wyeth company in USA acted very differently by giving us large quantities of injectible synthetic cyclic somatostatin with no strings attached.

We felt we had to try it out in ourselves and drew lots, Lundbæk indicated a wish to participate, but accepted our argument that the possible loss to mankind and science was too great. I won and felt as probably the first human being the bradycardia lasting about one minute after the intravenous injection of 500 µg somatostatin.

After this encouragement, we injected it in the rest of us five and in a few type 1 diabetes patients just before an exercise stimulation test. We noted marked growth hormone suppression in all [16]. As an unbelievable extra bonus, we stumbled over the first discovered extrapituitary effect of somatostatin: inhibition of insulin secretion [17]. All this happened thanks to Wyeth within the year of the discovery of somatostatin, 1973.

But somatostatin was not to give the desired final validation of our theory, nor to become the compound to combat proliferative retinopathy. Firstly due to its numerous other effects, and primarily because of its terrific short half life. As we stated later, future trials would require an analogue with more specific growth hormone inhibitory action as well as a much more protracted action.

The latter goal was partly achieved with Sandoz' development of the analogue octreotide (Sandostatin).

Kierkegaard et al and Nørgaard et al [18, 19] performed a controlled clinical study of effects in type 1 diabetic patients, who for one year received continuous subcutaneous infusion of octreotide or placebo.

It had for years been impossible to consider experiments in patients with proliferative retinopathy, so the study was restricted to patients with background retinopathy. It did not demonstrate any differences in progress of angiopathy in the two relatively small groups during the relatively short intervention. A further obstacle may have been that pituitary ablation had only had effect in cases with proliferative retinopathy, never in patients with background retinopathy.

This unrivalled study followed and was followed by a number of uncontrolled ones and casuistic reports, most of which had been unduly optimistic.

It had finally become evident that future studies must include a large number of patients in proper randomized controlled trials treated for several years with a somatostatin analogue or placebo and then observe the incidence of worsening of their background retinopathy.

Novartis initiated such a large multicentre study in hundreds of patients treated once monthly with very long acting octreotide (*Sandostatin® LAR®*). The study was closed recently after 3 to 5 years, but no results have yet been published.

Including IGF-I

It was obvious to investigate whether IGF-I, the mediator of growth hormone's growth effects, had any role in the proliferative vascular manifestations.

Plasma IGF-I is primarily produced in the liver and is a true hormone with universal mitogenic effects. It is as mentioned upon low in type 1 diabetic patients, probably due to hepatic resistance to growth hormone, which again is caused by portal insulinopenia.

But IGF-I is also produced in all organs that may be stricken by diabetic angiopathy and acts in an autocrine/paracrine manner. It is not yet established whether these *local* peripheral production sites are also resistant to the diabetic hypersomatotropinaemia.

The vast majority of clinical studies have concerned evaluation of the *circulating IGF-I's* possible role in diabetic angiopathy and been inconclusive.

Abnormalities in *local* IGF-I are almost always impossible to ascertain in clinical studies. An exception is an attempt to evaluate IGF-I determinations in fluid obtained after vitrectomies. Elevated levels were reported in diabetes patients compared to controls, but the whole situation is so complex, and avoidance of contamination with blood so difficult, that the conclusions must be assessed with caution.

We have studied renal IGF-I in experimental diabetes in rats and found that a local accumulation took place during the first two days after diabetes induction just before the well-known kidney hypertrophy started [20].

Both could be prevented by insulin as well as octreotide administration [21]. More relevant from the view point of long-term nephropathy, we found that octreotide given twice daily for half a year prevented the huge increase in albumiuria in diabetic rats and reduced histological manifestations [22].

Allan Flyvbjerg et al extended these findings to include growth hormone deficient rats, as well as by long-term administration of the specific growth hormone receptor antagonist pegvisomant with similar outcome. This study gave strong evidence that local IGF-I in contrast to liver IGF-I was sensitive to the growth hormone hypersecretion [23].

In conclusion, the growth hormone hypothesis has survived for 38 years, it has been slightly extended to include macroangiopathy and a role for IGF-I, but the message is unchanged.

It is still regarded by many with scepticism, although all now acknowledge that normal weight diabetes patients hypersecrete growth hormone throughout their life in a magnitude inversely dependent on their metabolic control. And those who have perused Sharp et al's follow-up study (10) will accept that pituitary ablation protected the diabetic eye from worsening of proliferative retinopathy at least as effectively as the later introduced photocoagulation. However, hypophysectomy is a serious interference, acutely, as well as after the operation, particularly in fragile long-term diabetes patients, who become excessively sensitive to insulin. So it was with marked relief, when it was succeeded by laser photocoagulation.

We realise of course that growth hormone and IGF-I are not the only players, and that others must participate. In our biased eyes these putative factors are not more firmly established. In brief, the growth hormone hypothesis is thus at present neither discarded nor finally proven.

Acknowledgments

I wish to thank all the members of successive teams, who dreamed up the projects – and first of all the technicians who accomplished that some of the fantasies became real.

REFERENCES

1. *Lundbæk K, Jensen VA, Olsen ST, Ørskov H, Christensen NJ, Johansen K, Hansen AP, Østerby R. Diabetes, diabetic angiopathy, and growth hormone. Lancet 1970;II:131-3*
2. *Lundbæk K. Long-term diabetes. – The clinical picture in diabetes mellitus of 15-25 years duration, with a follow-up of a regional series of cases. (The ophtalmological section in collaboration with V.A. Jensen). Monograph. Copenhagen: Munksgaard, 1953*
3. *Lundbæk K, Diabetic angiopathy – a specific vascular disease. Lancet 1954;I:377-9*
4. *Poulsen JD. Diabetes and anterior pituitary deficiency. Diabetes 1953;2:7-12*
5. *Yde H. The growth hormone dependent sulfation factor in serum from patients with various types of diabetes. Acta Med Scand 1969;186:293-7.*
6. *Ørskov H, Thomsen HG, Yde H. Wick-chromatography for rapid and reliable immunoassay of insulin, glucagon and growth hormone. Nature 1968;219:193-7*
7. *Hansen AP. Abnormal serum growth hormone response to exercise in juvenile diabetics. J Clin Invest 1970;49:1476-87*

8. Hansen AP. Normalisation of growth hormone response to exercise in juvenile diabetics. J Clin Invest 1971;50:1806-11
9. Ledet T. Growth hormone antiserum suppresses the growth effect of diabetic serum. Diabetes 1977;26:798-803
10. Sharp PS, Fallon TJ, Brazier J, Sandler LM, Joplin GF, Kohner EM. Long term follow-up of patients who underwent yttrium-90 pituitary implantation for treatment of proliferative diabetic retinopathy. Diabetologia 1987;30:199-207
11. Deckert T, Simonsen E, Poulsen JE. Prognosis for vision in proliferative retinopathy in juvenile diabetes. Diabetes 1967;728-33
12. Sharp P. Diabetic retinopathy: An analysis of the possible pathogenic roles of growth hormone and insulin-like growth factor I. In: Flyvbjerg A, Ørskov H, Alberti KGMM, eds. Growth Hormone and Insulin-like growth factor I in Human and Experimental Diabetes. Chichester: John Wiley & Sons, 1993:204-28
13. Merimee TJ, Fineberg, SE, Mckusick VA, Hall J. Diabetes mellitus and sexual ateliotic dwarfism: a comparative study. J Clin Invest 1970;49:1096-102
14. Merimee TJ. A follow-up study of vascular disease in growth hormone deficient dwarfs with diabetes. N Engl J Med 1978;298:1217-22
15. Brazeau P, Vale W, Burgus R, Ling N, Butcher M, Rivier J, Guillemin R. Hypothalamic peptide that inhibits the secretion of immunoreactive pituitary growth hormone. Science 1973;179:77-9
16. Hansen AP, Ørskov H, Seyer-Hansen K, Lundbæk K. Some actions of growth hormone release inhibiting factor. Br Med J 1973;3:523-4
17. Alberti KGMM, Christensen SE, Christensen NJ, Hansen AP, Iversen J, Lundbæk K, Seyer-Hansen K, Ørskov H. Inhibition of insulin secretion by somatostatin. (Citation Classic, Current Contents, 1982). Lancet 1973; II:1299-301
18. Kierkegaard C, Nørgaard K, Snorgaard O, Bek T, Lassen M, Lund Andersen H. Effect of one year continuous subcutaneous infusion of a somatostatin analogue, octreotide, on early retinopathy, metabolic control and thyroid function in type I (insulin dependent) diabetes mellitus. Acta Endocrinol (Copenh)1990;122:766-72
19. Nørgaard K, Snorgaard T, Jensen T, Kierkegaard C. Effects of octreotide on lipoproteins and endothelial function in type I (insulin dependent) diabetic patients. Diabet Med 1990;7:909-13
20. Flyvbjerg A, Thorlacius-Ussing O, Næraa R, Ingerslev J, Ørskov H. Kidney tissue somatomedin C and initial renal growth in diabetic and uninephrectomized rats. Diabetologia 1988;31:310-4
21. Flyvbjerg A, Frystyk J, Thorlacius-Ussing O, Ørskov H. Somatostatin analogue administration prevents increase in kidney somatomedin C and ini-

tial renal growth in diabetic and uninephrectomized rats. Diabetologia 1989;32:261–5

22. *Flyvbjerg A, Marshall SM, Frystyk J, Hansen KW, Harris A.G., Ørskov H. Octreotide administration in diabetic rats: Effect on kidney growth and urinary albumin excretion. Kidney Int 1992;41:805–12*
23. *Flyvbjerg A, Bennett WF, Rasch R, Kopchick JJ, Scharlett JA. Inhibitory effect of a growth hormone receptor antagonist. (G120K–PEG) on renal enlargement, glomerular hypertrophy and urinary albumin excretion on experimental diabetes in mice. Diabetes 1999;48:377–82*

NEPHROPATHY – THE LONG ROAD FROM IDEA TO PREVENTION

CARL ERIK MOGENSEN

The mentor and his importance

Knud Lundbæk, the world famous diabetologist, for many years professor of internal medicine at the University of Aarhus, Department of Medicine M, introduced me to diabetology, and of course I still regard him as my mentor. The idea of prevention in connection with diabetic nephropathy was, to put it mildly, not particularly clear, when at one point in 1964 as a student of medicine I cautiously approached Knud Lundbæk and expressed my interest in doing medical research. The idea of working under Knud Lundbæk came from my study mate and good colleague for many years, Thomas Ledet, who was already at that time engaged in writing a University Medal thesis. It was a really exciting period in the years around 1970 with the production of many DMSc dissertations from Department M.

Lundbæk was the leading figure and source of inspiration, also for me. In addition, I received really good help in the laboratory, especially from Hans Ørskov along with Hans Jørgen Gundersen. Hans Ørskov was and is unique, also in the laboratory as a helper and source of inspiration with a view to introducing new ideas and methods. Thus, he was one of the first to use radioimmunoassays in Denmark. Hans Jørgen Gundersen was of great assistance with his knowledge of statistics and his laboratory techniques. However, the starting point for my studies was a cooperation with Ruth Østerby.

Knud Lundbæk investigated diabetic angiopathy from various angles, and he also introduced the term "late diabetes" or "long-term diabetes" [1]. It was therefore a provocation that Marvin Siperstein from Texas published data [2] obtained by electron microscopy on muscle biopsies, measurements that indicated blood vessel lesions already at the start of the disease. He wrote: "*These results indicate that thickening of the muscle capillary basement membranes is a characteristic of genetic diabetes mellitus, and further, that the hyperglycemia of diabetes is probably not the factor responsible for the microangiopathy characteristic of diabetes mellitus".* Genetic predisposition was the prevalent concept for many years in the USA, where many diabetologists headed by E Tolstoj in New York [3], believed that good glucose regulation for diabetes patients was not particularly relevant. In opposition to this view, the Joslin Diabetes Center argued for good diabetes regulation, but it was incomparably easier to accept a not particularly good regulation when treating patients. It apparently made life easier for them in the short term, and it was believed that there were no convincing studies indicating that good regulation had any real effect on the development of blood vessel, nerve and kidney lesions. In contrast, it was the prevalent view in Europe that good metabolic regulation was essential. Here it was thought that the genetic element was of minor importance. It was therefore extra provocative that Siperstein proposed that there was a very strong genetic element in the genesis of complications [2]. In Lundbæk's opinion, this was based on unreliable results deriving from muscle biopsies, in which it is difficult to obtain precise figures.

Kidney biopsy/kidney function

This gave Lundbæk the idea of investigating the kidney's glomeruli in newly diagnosed type 1 diabetes. That is to say that kidney biopsies were taken for patients with newly diagnosed type 1 diabetes, and these were repeated some years later. Ruth Østerby was the person who would introduce morphometry into diabetology [4]. It is well known that she did not find structural measurable changes in the basal membrane, especially in the thickness of the basal membrane in newly diagnosed type 1 diabetes. This was an important argument indicating that kidney and vessel lesions came secondarily in connection with diabetes, even though patients with newly diagnosed diabetes have hyperfiltration and large kidneys [5].

My role as a medical student was to find a functional correlation to the structural changes in the kidney. Lundbæk had just been on a lecture trip to England, where he met John Hardwicke. The latter had introduced dextran clearance determinations for patients with proteinuria with a view to exactly defining the glomerular permeability for macromolecules.

It was my task with this technique to assess the glomerular function in healthy persons and in patients with diabetes mellitus, including both patients with short-term – and thereby newly diagnosed diabetes – and long-term diabetes, as well as in patients with and without complications [5]. It did not prove possible to find convincing signs of change in the glomerular permeability with dextran clearance, when it was expressed as a percentage of the glomerular filtration rate (GFR). The difficulties with GFR data were thus a central problem. I therefore set about inulin clear-

Studies related to nephromegaly, hyperfiltration, microalbuminuria, glomerulopathy, epidemiology, metabolic syndrome, and significance of near-normal glycaemia

Phenomenon	Nephromegaly	Hyperfiltration	Immune-measurement of urinary albumin
Early observation	Paris, 1849 C. Bernard	Italy, Switzerland 1950-1960	Uppsala, 1961
Subsequent studies and observations	Several pathologists (but not carefully documented)	Denmark, 1970	London, 1963
Newer studies	Aarhus, 1973 Copenhagen, 1991	Minneapolis, predictive of microalbuminuria. Aarhus, 1984 UK, USA, Sweden, Italy 2005	Aarhus, 1970
Confirmed and/or clinical significant	Munich, 1998 Milan, 2006 predictive of renal disease – not clinically used	Clinical assessment may be problematic	Rapid procedures Aarhus, 1995, w used

The concept of renoprotection. Physiological and genetic studies in diabetes

Phenomenon	Protection by AHT. Incipient nephropathy (type 1)	Protection by AHT. Overt nephropathy (type 1)	Protection by AHT in microalb. (type 1)	ACE-I and renal protection
Early observation	Aarhus, 1985 Copenhagen Melbourne Paris	Aarhus, 1976-82 CPH, 1983 Gothenburg	Aarhus	Aarhus, Paris Copenhagen Melbourne
Newer studies	Aarhus Italy Copenhagen	Many studies	Several studies	UKPDS (probably similar effect with beta-blockers)
Confirmed and/or clinical significant	Several guidelines	Several guidelines	Multifactorial intervention important	Maybe more effective than ordinary AHT

ʍicroalbuminuria T1DM	Glomerulopathy and proteinuria	Epidemiology of microalb. and mortality, incl. T2DM	The metabolic syndrome	Significance of glycaemic control
.ondon, 1964 ˢarhus, 1971	Kimmelstiel and Wilson, 1936	London, 1964 epidemiology Aarhus, 1983, mortality	Sweden, 1923 England, 1939 France, 1949 Italy, 1965	Keiding, 1952 proving the concept Pirart 1978
ollow-up: .ondon, 1982 CPH, 1982 arhus, 1984	Several pathologists, e.g. Gellman, 1959	Aarhus Fredericia London	Ferranini Reaven Hoorn Study	Scandinavia Gothenburg Kumamoto
Many studies	Aarhus Minneapolis (morphometry), 1965	Mortality data firmly confirmed in meta-analysis	Concept used by many investigators, but correlation not too close	DCCT Oslo/Aarhus UKPDS
nportant guidelines. Cyclosporine results in enal damage Gentofte)	Several reviews Biopsy rarely needed	Used now in all epidemiological and large trials	Still variations in definition. One element requires screening for the other risks	Several guidelines (widely accepted, but AHT may be equally important or more)

omplications enetically etermined?	Provocation tests (e.g. exercise)	24 h amb. BP in diabetes	Dextran Ficoll and polyvinyl clearance	Dual blockade of RAS in diabetes
iperstein, 1973, eckert, Gentofte, ondon oston CPH rance	Karlefors Aarhus	Rubler Aarhus	Uppsala Düsseldorf Aarhus Liège	Aarhus, 2000 CPH, 2002-2006
omplications netabolically etermined and nodulated by ypertension	Only few studies	Several studies	CPH San Francisco	Positive studies, also in non-diabetics
Metabolic control ssential	Not used, but may be relevant in treatment trials	Of great value and should be used more clinically	Groningen. Not used any longer	May be used when BP-control is difficult

ance in order to get an exact measurement of GFR. Surprisingly, it turned out that patients with newly diagnosed type 1 diabetes had abnormally high GFR, that is, so-called hyperfiltration. This had been previously described, but it has always been a paradox that patients who later lost their kidney function because of diabetes had initially had hyperfiltration [5-10].

Early hyperfiltration – and subsequent fall in GFR

The concept of "hyperfiltration" was first introduced from a theoretical and animal-experimental angle by Barry Brenner [11]. He found that hyperfiltration was a marked pathogenetic mechanism in the development of renal disease, especially in an experimental situation with a varying degree of nephrectomy (removal of the kidney). We were able to document that hyperfiltration was a function of the metabolic regulation, inasmuch as GFR fell with long-term good blood glucose regulation introduced in connection with newly diagnosed diabetes mellitus. Acute fluctuations in blood glucose did not give variation in kidney function. Furthermore, most diabetes patients, who were of course not particularly well regulated, had a somewhat higher GFR than the background population, and while healthy young persons as a rule had a GFR of between 110 and 120 ml/min/1.73m^2, the typical diabetes patient had a GFR of 140. For poorly regulated diabetes or newly diagnosed diabetes GFR was often 170 ml/min/1.73 m^2. Similar findings were made by Jørn Ditzel from Aalborg. Reviewing the literature, one can be in no doubt that this was a marked and correct finding way back in European studies, an observation that had thus become of topical significance. Also the tubular function measured as the kidney's absorption of glucose was found to be increased [5].

We knew early on that hyperfiltration seemed to be a risk factor – the higher the GFR, the higher the risk of developing initial and manifest renal disease. This evoked a good deal of criticism from England and the USA, but the results have later been confirmed in comprehensive studies from England, the USA and Italy [6, 7]. The question was now when and how the fall in GFR starts in type 1 diabetes – a fall that sooner or later ends in a total cessation of the renal function in some patients (today fortunately fewer and fewer). Our investigations showed that even patients with long-term diabetes without proteinuria in fact had a well preserved renal function with GFR of around 140. By examining patients with proteinuria prospectively, on the other hand, there proved to be a marked fall in GFR when they were examined every six months or once a year with a precise technique. I was thus able to define the rate of reduction in GFR, which was on average about 1 ml/min/month with proteinuria, albeit with large variations.

The pivotal idea: early blood pressure treatment

It was furthermore an important observation that a high blood pressure level correlated strongly with the fall in renal function. This was an interesting observation, as it could indicate that treatment with blood pressure lowering medicine could reduce the rate of fall in GFR.

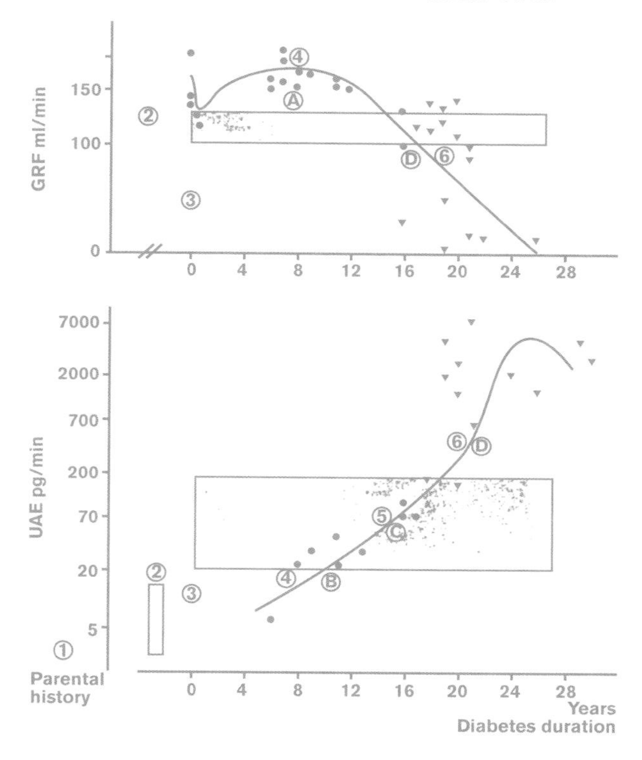

Prediction and treatment of diabetic renal disease in patients with type 1 diabetes. GFR = Glomerular filtration rate; UAE = Urinary albumin excretion rate. Predictors: ① Genetics in relation to diabetic renal disease is still a "big black hole"; ② On diagnosis of diabetes, blood pressure is a little higher in patients with subsequent microalbuminuria (not HbA_{1c} *or C-peptide); ③–④ Albumin secretion rate is a little higher with subsequent microalbuminuria. Isolated hyperfiltration and higher* HbA_{1c} *are predictive risk factors for microalbuminuria, as is increased thickening of basal membrane. ⑤–⑥ Higher blood pressure and poor glycaemic control accelerate albuminuria and the fall in GFR. Antihypertensive treatment required. Intervention: Ⓐ–Ⓑ Close to normal albumin secretion; Ⓒ Early lowering of blood pressure inhibits progression to proteinuria; Ⓓ Effective antihypertensive treatment reduces the fall in GFR. (Commentaries on Perspectives in Diabetes, vol. 1, 1988–92, American Diabetes Association, and Diabetes Mellitus, vol. IV, Garland).*

This was a completely new concept. Earlier it had been thought that it was necessary to have a certain blood pressure level in order to ensure renal perfusion (flushing of the kidney). In fact, that is said to be the background for the term "essential hypertension", which suggests that it is necessary to have a certain increase in blood pressure in order to ensure perfusion of various organs, especially the kidney. This would, however, prove to be a decidedly erroneous view. A change of paradigm was initiated in which the leading principle was to lower blood pressure in order to preserve the renal function.

I actually performed the very first studies in this regard [12]. Furthermore, it turned out that increased blood pressure was a marked risk factor for cardiovascular disorders. Blood pressure treatment is thus effective with a view to preventing cardiovascular disorders. It was extremely exciting to be at the centre of such a change of paradigm, which proved to exert an extremely marked influence on the research of the following decades – right up to 2007. It was necessary not to be confused by the fact that blood pressure lowering treatment had an initial and slightly reducing effect on GFR. This is merely a reflection of the physiological mechanism: a fall in transglomerular pressure.

It also proved to be the case that in short-term studies blood pressure treatment had a marked effect on the secretion of albumin in the urine. The short-term effect on albumin secretion apparently correlated with the blood pressure effect. This could indicate a long-term favourable effect on the fall rate in GFR, which has later been confirmed.

The results of the blood pressure treatment on the renal function [12] were first presented at the so-called Kroc Foundation Meetings in California. Two meetings were held.

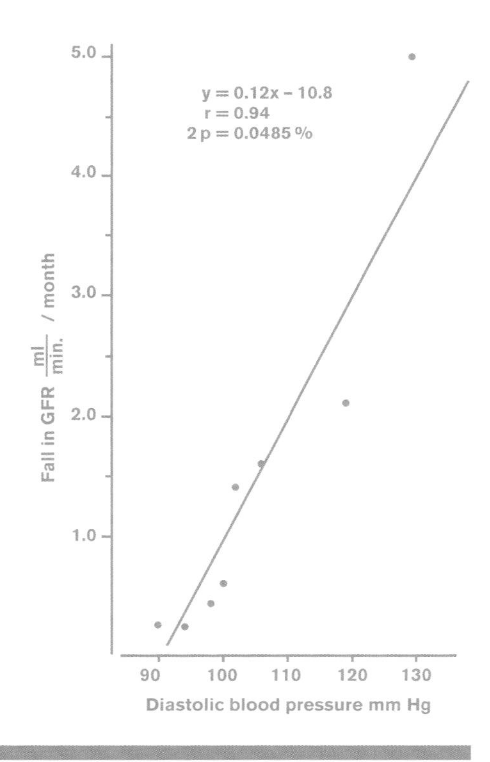

The fall in the glomerular filtration rate (GFR) is correlated with the diastolic blood pressure. (Data from author).

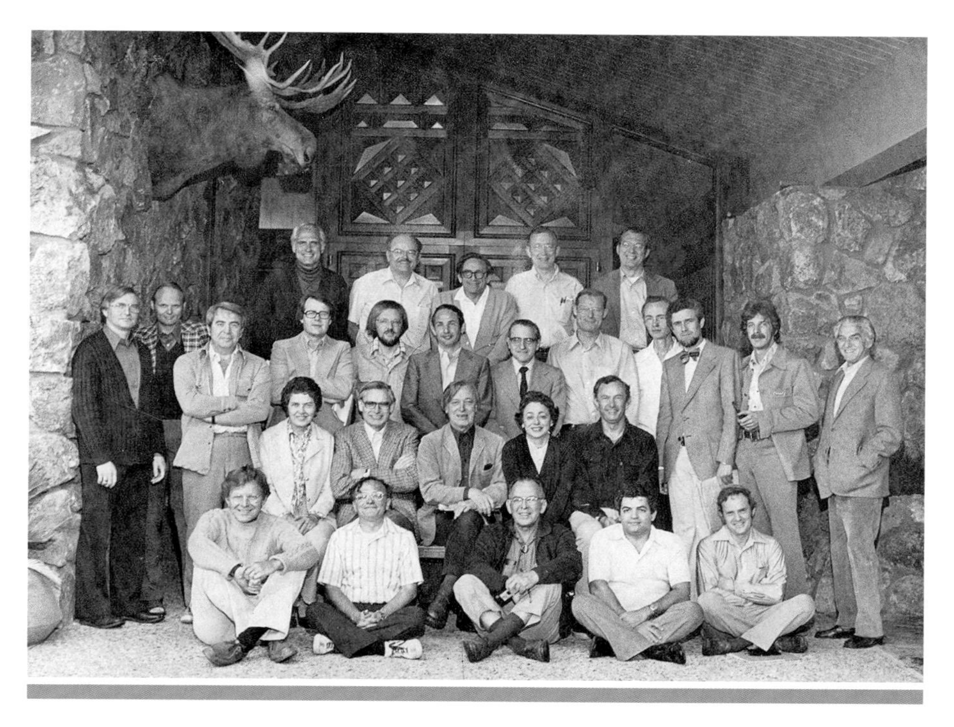

Participants in the Kroc Foundation's first diabetes meeting in 1976.

The first in 1976 and the second in 1982. Hans-Henrik Parving also participated in the first Kroc meeting. He reported on transcapillary passage of albumin [13] in diabetes mellitus and was well acquainted with my studies of glycaemic regulation and albumin secretion. On the plane on the way home, he was really enthusiastic about our new results: the positive effect of blood pressure treatment. He wished to test and possibly reproduce these results on a larger material, which was available at Hvidøre and later at Steno Diabetes Center. Parving's first results were then presented at the next Kroc meeting in 1982, and at this time, I had follow-up data covering a lengthy period. My results were soon after published in the British Medical Journal, also in 1982 [14]. The road to prevention thus starts in 1976 or thereabouts. But the general dissemination of the idea probably gained ground only around the end of the 1980s and in the beginning of the 1990s. When outpatient blood pressure registration became technically possible, a 24-hour blood pressure registration showed a considerably better correlation to albuminuria and renal function changes than hitherto, while it was also possible to describe changes in 24-hour variations.

It is still being discussed, and rightly so, to what extent the effect has to do with the blood pressure treatment alone or is specially related to blocking of the renin-angiotensin system. I found a marked effect from diuretics and beta blockade, which was later reproduced by Parving. There is probably general agreement that blood pressure treatment is clearly the most important element, but it is likely that there is a secondary gain to be had from using substances that inhibit the renin-angiotensin system. At any rate, this has a pronounced effect on the proteinuria or albuminuria and possibly also on the hyperfiltration, as we found in studies with angiogenesis II receptor blocker preparations (ARBs). As is well known, results achieved in Europe (also the miroalbuminuria idea, for example) have rarely gained acceptance in the USA before they have been reproduced there. This was the case for the so-called *Captopril®* study of nephropathy in type 1 diabetes, where there was an effect of the treatment (with clear reference to our studies 10 years earlier) [10]. New meta-analyses show that the positive effect on GFR is clearly relevant in relation to the fall in blood pressure. Dual blockade, i.e. blockade of both ACE and angiogenesis receptor, may be relevant if the blood pressure cannot be controlled in other ways. For diabetes this was documented in our CALM study in a controlled clinical investigation with positive effect on patients with type 2 diabetes and microalbuminuria [15]. These studies were confirmed by Parving and greatly elaborated by Parving and colleagues.

An impressive series of ground-breaking studies have since been carried out by Professor Hans-Henrik Parving and his colleagues [15-16]. A large number of DMSc dissertations have been completed in continuation of a line of research set out by Torsten Deckert and later by Oluf Pedersen. A number of DMSc dissertations and PhD theses have also come from Århus.

Microalbuminuria – a new concept

To identify patients who develop proteinuria, we conducted long-term investigations of GFR and albumin secretion. It soon became clear that increased albumin secretion that was beneath the proteinuria level was a risk factor for development of manifest renal disease and thus a marked risk factor [9]. Together with colleagues in Gentofte and London, we therefore introduced the concept of "microalbuminuria" [17]. Not only is microalbuminuria an important risk factor for the development of renal disease, but studies subsequently showed that like proteinuria microalbuminuria constituted a considerable risk of mortality and cardiovascular disease in patients with both type 1 and type 2 diabetes as well as in the background population (this was documented in our Fredericia study).

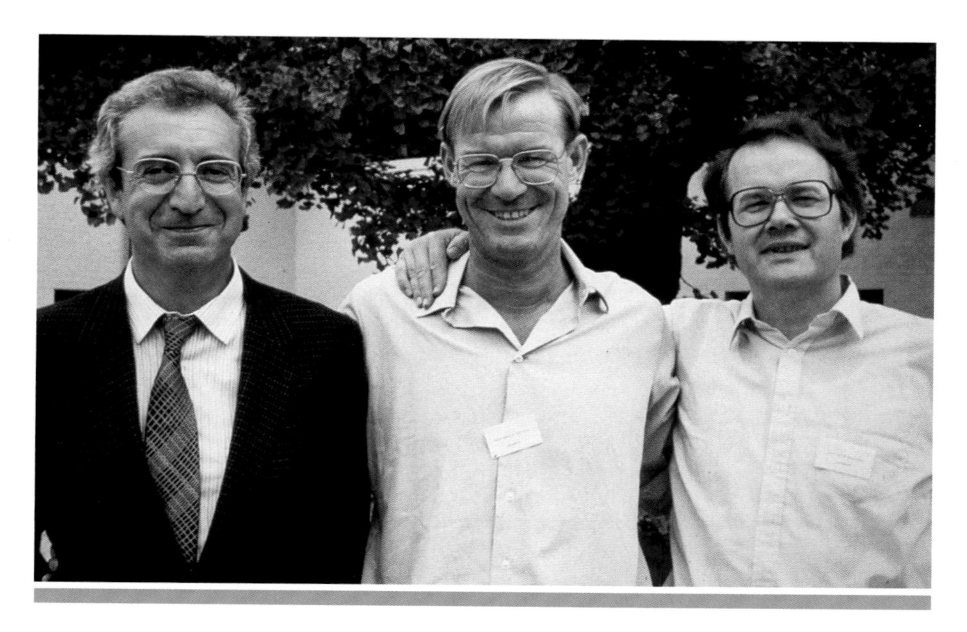

The three gentlemen who defined microalbuminuria. From the left: GC Viberti, Hans-Henrik Parving and Carl Erik Mogensen.

The problem in treating patients with manifest renal disease was that although one could reduce the fall rate for GFR, one could not stop the fall completely. In order to prevent manifest renal disease, it therefore became relevant to define patients with microalbuminuria somewhat more precisely. We were able to show that these patients often have a well preserved renal function, and even still have hyperfiltration. It was therefore relevant to start antihypertensive treatment for these patients, even though their blood pressure was only marginally increased. We examined and treated the type 1 diabetes patients irrespective of blood pressure level and monitored GFR and abumin secretion before and after treatment [10]. The first studies were performed with beta blockers and diuretics and showed positive results. Hypoglycaemia could be a risk factor when treating these patients with beta blockers. Mathiesen followed up quickly by using the ACE inhibitor *Captopril®* for patients with microalbuminuria and confirmed that a fall in GFR could be prevented or reduced [10].

The ACE inhibitors were not involved in the development of hypoglycaemia, but had a good effect in patients with diabetes mellitus through a general lowering of their blood pressure and the pressure over the glomerulus membrane. This led to a breakthrough in the prevention of diabetic renal disease. Similar studies also came from Michel Marre in France, from our group and from Steno Diabetes Center [16]. Østerby was able to document that the structural changes were stabilized by treatment of blood pressure with both beta blockers and ACE inhibitors [10].

Thus, one can say that some marked risk factors such as albuminuria, microalbuminuria and high blood pressure have been described. The clinical process has been described reasonably thoroughly, and an association between blood pressure and the progression of renal disease has been found. With an effective treatment, we are well on the way towards effective prevention and treatment. Perhaps one could call it a medical hat trick.

Theory of science and guidelines

Numerous guidelines have appeared in the wake of these studies, and in retrospect, it has been extremely interesting to have been part of this process.

One could also reflect on theories of science. At courses in this discipline, one learns that one must put forward a hypothesis and try to confirm or invalidate it. This has in part also been the case in the study of diabetic renal disease, although it must be said that naturally the ideas have appeared in the course of research, just as one's appetite perhaps comes while one is

Problematic and non-topical additions concerning kidney and diabetes		**The author's assessment**
1)	Genetic analysis relevant in connection with risk assessment, diagnosis and treatment	Not documented yet
2)	High blood pressure relevant to secure kidney perfusion	Historically interesting, but a misunderstanding
3)	Renal biopsy relevant with a view to diagnosing non-diabetic nephropathy in type 1 and type 2 diabetes patients (not in connection with absence of retinopathy)	Renal biopsy very rarely required
4)	Protein-reduced diet useful concerning inhibition of progression of diabetic renal disease, also in ACE-I and ARB treatment	Protein reduction does not affect the fall in GFR in connection with ACE-inhibitors/ARBs
5)	Angiotensin receptor blockers (ARBs) always first choice for type 2 diabetes and microalbuminuria/light albuminuria	Both ACE-inhibitors and ARB scan be used
6)	Use of contraceptive pill associated with future nephropathy	Not confirmed in major studies in the USA

eating. A result brings with it a new question, which must in its turn be answered until one possibly arrives at ideas and programmes for treatment that can benefit the patients effectively. One might also say that one hypothesis follows the other [18-20].

Genetics

If we return to our point of departure, which was that a number of Americans very decidedly asserted that genetics was the key factor, it must be said that reliable genetic markers for diabetic renal disease have still not been found, even though a combination of markers might possibly be relevant. But we are still in suspense awaiting these results. On the other hand, as described in the Steno 2 study, it is the treatment of the known risk factors that is of crucial importance [10]. However, the treatment programmes presented are not totally sufficient with a view to the patients attaining a normal life span. The question therefore still remains open for discussion: *"Complications, fault or destiny?"*

Conclusion

As will have appeared from the foregoing, Denmark has played an important role in the investigation, prevention and treatment of diabetic nephropathy. This also appears from the bibliometric data, but a complete bibliometric assessment that comprises number of publications, number of citations, originality, impact factor of journals and the like has not yet been generally accepted [18]. The studies that have been published in this field from our small country therefore continue to be subject to the unconstrained judgements of others [18].

REFERENCES

1. *Lundbæk K. Long-term diabetes. The clinical picture in diabetes mellitus of 15-25 years' duration with a follow-up of a regional series of cases. Copenhagen: Munksgaard; London, New York: Lange, Maxwell & Springer, 1953*

2. Siperstein MD, Unger RH, Madison LL. Studies of muscle capillary basement membranes in normal subjects, diabetic, and prediabetic patients. J Clin Invest 1968;47:1973-99
3. Ricketts HT. Does hyperglycemia harm the diabetic patient? The Medical Clinics of North America. Philadelphia and London: W.B. Saunders Company, 1947:267-78
4. Østerby R. Early phases in the development of diabetic glomerulopathy. A quantitative electron microscopic study. Acta Med Scand 1975;Suppl. 574:1-82
5. Mogensen CE. Hyperfiltration, hypertension, and diabetic nephropathy in IDDM patients. Based on the Golgi Lecture 1988, EASD Meeting, Paris. Diabetes Nutr Metab 1989;2:227-44
6. Mogensen CE. Prediction of clinical diabetic nephropathy in IDDM patients. Alternatives to microalbuminuria? Diabetes 1990:39;761-7
7. Mogensen CE. Prediction of clinical diabetic nephropathy in Type 1 diabetic patients: Alternatives to microalbuminuria? Messages related to the microalbuminuria concept: 1990-2006. In: Robertson RP, ed. Commentaries on perspectives in diabetes, ADA 2006:116-122
8. Mogensen CE. Diabetic renal disease: The quest for normotension – and beyond. Diabet Med 1995;12:756-69
9. Mogensen CE. Microalbuminuria, blood pressure and diabetic renal disease: origin and development of ideas (based upon the Claude Bernard Lecture, 1998). Diabetologia 1999; 42:263-85
10. Mogensen CE. Microalbuminuria and hypertension with focus on type 1 and type 2 diabetes (based upon the Anders Jahre lecture). J Int Med 2003;254:45-66
11. Hostetter HT, Troy JL, Brenner BM. Glomerular hemodynamics in experimental diabetes mellitus. Kidney Int 1981;19:410-6
12. Mogensen CE. Renal function changes in diabetes. Diabetes 1976;25(suppl.2):872-9
13. Parving H-H. Increased microvascular permeability to plasma proteins in short- and long-term juvenile diabetes. Diabetes 1976;25(suppl.2):884-9
14. Mogensen CE. Long-term antihypertensive treatment inhibiting progression of diabetic nephropathy. Br Med J 1982;285:685-8
15. Mogensen CE, Andersen NH. Diabetic renal and related heart disease. ACE-inhibitors and/or angiotensin receptor blockers: does it matter? In: Cortes P, Mogensen CE, eds. Contemporary Diabetes: The Diabetic Kidney. Totowa, NJ: Humana Press, 2006:437-51
16. Rossing P. Prediction, progression and prevention of diabetic nephropathy. The Minkowski Lecture 2005. Diabetologia 2006;49:11-9
17. Mogensen CE, Chacati A, Christensen CK, Close CF, Deckert T, Hommel E, Kastrup J, Lefebvre P, Mathiesen ER, Feldt-Rasmussen B. Microalbu-

minuria: An early marker of renal involvement in diabetes. Uremia Invest 1985-1986;9:85-95

18. *Hirsch JE. An index to quantify an individual's scientific research output. Proc Natl Acad Sci U S A 2005;102:16569-72*
19. *Hall PH. Prevention of progression in diabetic nephropathy. Diabetes Spectr 2006;19:18-24*
20. *Mogensen CE. Pathophysiology of diabetic complications. Abnormal physiological processes in kidney. In: Brownlee M, ed. Handbook of Diabetes, vol. 4: Biochemical Pathology. New York, London: Garland STPM Press, 1981:23-85*

DIABETES AND PREGNANCY

LARS MØLSTED-PEDERSEN

Before insulin came into clinical use in the beginning of the 1920s, very few women with diabetes became pregnant. For those who did become pregnant, the process was often fatal for both mother and infant. Maternal mortality was around 40 % and infant mortality was as high as almost 60 %.

With insulin treatment, the number of women in the childbearing age increased at the same time as their ability to become pregnant also increased. Maternal mortality for diabetes patients fell dramatically, while infant mortality remained high.

As registrar at Steno Memorial Hospital in the mid-1940s, Jørgen Pedersen – later professor of internal medicine at the University of Copenhagen – was interested by certain reports of pregnancy in diabetes patients [1]. In connection with his later appointment to Rigshospitalet's Maternity Unit, the "Centre for Pregnant Diabetics" was established in 1946 at Rigshospitalet, Copenhagen. The aim was through a clinical and scientific focus to reduce the high infant mortality (approx 40 %) late in pregnancy, during birth and just afterwards. This was a pioneering effort by a highly motivated personality with a great drive, who at an early stage placed Denmark in a leading position in this field.

Background

The diabetic metabolism becomes unstable during pregnancy, birth and the post-gestational period. As examples of typical fluctuations can be mentioned a tendency for low blood glucose (hypoglycaemia and insulin episodes) around the 10th week of pregnancy, the opposite – too high blood glucose (hyperglycaemia, ketoacidosis, diabetic coma) in weeks 26-30, and finally a strongly reduced insulin requirement as soon as the birth has taken place. After the middle of the pregnancy period, there is a pronounced deterioration of the diabetic metabolism – pregnancy has a diabetogenic effect.

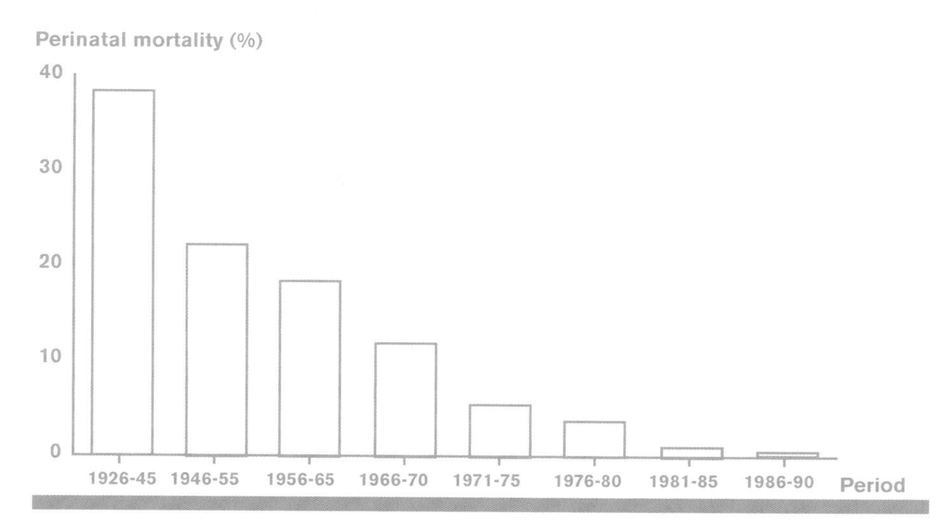

Perinatal mortality at Centre for Pregnant Diabetics, Rigshospitalet in children of mothers with diabetes. (Data from the author).

This appears, among other things, in the circumstance that approx 2 % of all pregnant women develop a, for the most part, mild diabetic condition during pregnancy named gestational diabetes (see below).

Seen from the obstetrician's viewpoint, the problems in the 1950s and 1960s were that the children had a tendency to die in the mother's womb during the last three weeks of pregnancy, and that some of the ordinary pregnancy complications like spontaneous premature birth (before week 37), pregnancy toxaemia, too much amniotic fluid and infection of the urinary tract were much more frequent than in mothers without diabetes.

The number of complications and the risk for the foetus were closely linked with the mother's diabetes regulation before and during pregnancy and furthermore with the mother's diabetes status prior to pregnancy (debut age and duration, diabetes-caused vascular changes especially in the eyes and kidneys). Priscilla White, a diabetologist from the Joslin Clinic in Boston, drew up a risk classification of pregnant diabetes patients on the basis of these variables. With her substantial contribution to the field of diabetes and pregnancy, she was both a pioneer and a source of inspiration for the treatment of these women [2].

Treatment

From the Centre's start, the main principles in the treatment have comprised:

- Centralisation of the treatment
- Cooperation between obstetrician, diabetologist and paediatrician
- Classification of the pregnancy
- Regulation of the diabetic metabolism
- Prevention and treatment of complications
- Careful planning, including setting the time and manner of the birth.

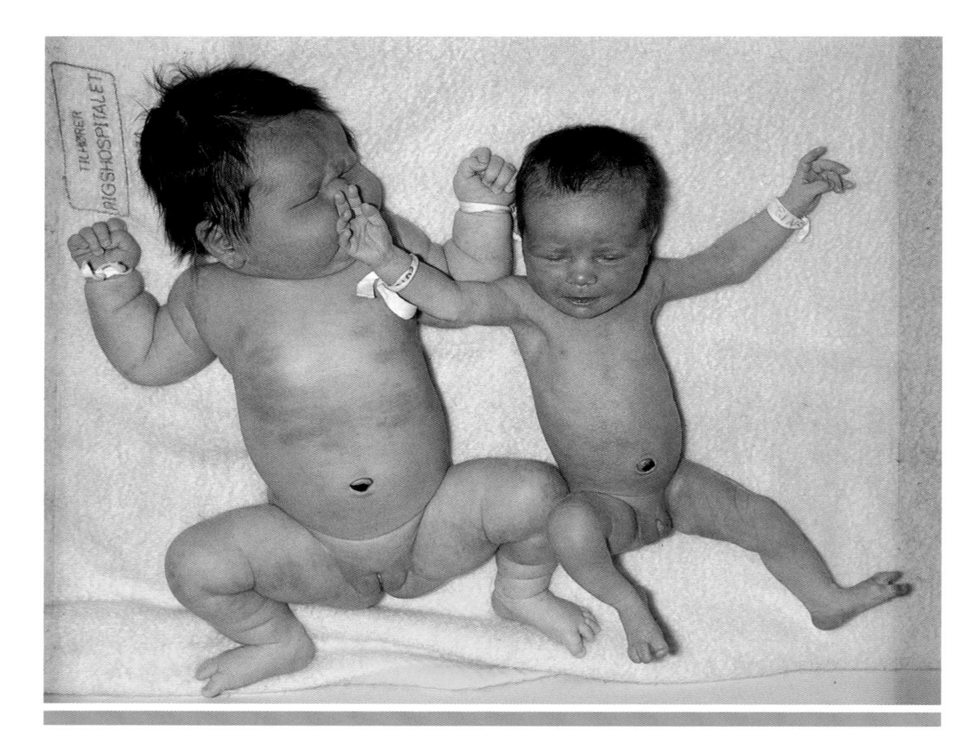

Two children born on the same day to diabetic mothers. Left: a far too large baby (4.700 g 54 cm), whose mother had diabetes for more than 10 years without eye complications. The mother's first contact with the centre was two days before the birth. Right: a too small baby (2.050 g, 44 cm). The mother had been followed by the centre throughout pregnancy, had both eye and kidney complications and slight pregnancy toxaemia (pre-eclampsia). Today by far the majority of babies are born with a normal weight.

In the first many years of the Centre's lifetime, the treatment was rather rigid and uniform for the entire patient group, and as this had yielded good results, it continued until the end of the 1970s. Patients were admitted for 4–6 days at the start of the pregnancy and then transferred to outpatient control approx. every two weeks and finally admitted 8 weeks preterm. As a rule, the birth was induced 3 weeks preterm. Discharge usually took place 8–10 days after birth.

It is often necessary to induce labour preterm, but on the other hand, the birth must not take place too early, for which there is a strong tendency in pregnant diabetes patients – both spontaneously and also because of complications. It is important to choose the right time for the birth, which in half of the patients takes place by caesarean section. In a survey from the Centre of 397 diabetic pregnancies from the period 1974–77, we found that infant mortality for the 65 % with a pregnancy of 37 weeks and more was very low (0.8 %), while the 35 % who had a shorter period of pregnancy had a perinatal mortality (infant mortality around the time of birth) of 12.2 % [3]. In recent years, the number of diabetes pregnancies of less than 37 weeks has fallen to under 20 %.

The decision as to the right time for a diabetes patient to give birth still requires great experience of the responsible obstetrician.

The rigid system has gradually been changed over the last 25–30 years. Today, the treatment has been individualized. For uncomplicated pregnant diabetes patients all pregnancy check-ups take place in the outpatients clinic, with the patients being seen by the same specialists in diabetology and obstetrics. The time of birth depends on the severity of the mother's diabetes, the size and wellbeing of the baby and on any pregnancy complications that might be present. On average, labour is induced medically, or a caesarean is performed, 8–10 days preterm for mothers with type 1 diabetes. The reason for this is that there is still no valid information as to whether these women can wait for a spontaneous birth at term without increased risk.

Pedersen and Brandstrup's demonstration in 1956 that a significant reduction in perinatal mortality (PM) was linked to how early the pregnant diabetes patients came under treatment at the Center led to this treatment being introduced in a number of other countries [4].

Diabetes and pregnancy as field of research

It was a surprise for all who were interested in the subject that the infant mortality in 1950 was as high as 40 %; the surviving children were a quite new population that had been exposed to a known, but pathological intrauterine environment with, among other things, too high blood glucose.

They presented a number of symptoms because of the ensuing hyperinsulinism. Insulin is the organism's dominant anabolic (tissue-building) hormone. When it is changed at the wrong time, the entire metabolism changes. By studying the mothers in pregnancy and the children after birth, one cannot only find treatment for their symptoms, but also contribute to increased knowledge about pregnancy and newborn infants.

Congenital malformations

I was inspired to interest myself in diabetes and pregnancy by Jørgen Pedersen, when I was appointed to Rigshospitalet's Maternity Unit in 1962. The perinatal mortality for diabetes pregnancies was 18 % in 1962. The major problem in these pregnancies was at this time severe congenital malformations. At an international level, it had not been definitively shown that there were more congenital malformations in children of diabetic mothers. In 1964, we clearly showed that this was the case, and furthermore we found a link between the diabetic vascular changes in the mother and the occurrence of severe congenital malformations in the child [5].

In 1977, once again we drew up accounts over the congenital malformations, and this time we divided the pregnant mothers into two groups: the diabetes patients who prior to pregnancy had been regulated at one of the two hospitals, Steno Memorial Hospital and Hvidøre Hospital, and the rest of those who had given birth in the period 1966–77. In the groups with many years of diabetes and/or vascular changes owing to diabetes, both the total number and the number of severe malformations were significantly lower in the Steno-Hvidøre group. These observations made us incline more towards a metabolic background for the malformations, while the theory of vascular complications as a cause of the malformations was weakened [6].

In September 1977, a young obstetrician from Greifswald in East Germany (DDR) took part in the Diabetic Pregnancy Study Group's meeting in Copenhagen, and as pregnant diabetes patients in the DDR were under good control, a joint project was agreed. The goal was to cooperate on comparing the occurrence of malformations in two groups with type 1 diabetes: a group that was well regulated prior to pregnancy with a group that did not come to control until after the 8th–10th week of pregnancy. However, we did not hear any more of the project despite writing several letters until the article was published exclusively with DDR figures in 1983 [7].

The theory has since proved to hold water: there is a significant link between the mother's blood glucose in the first weeks of pregnancy up to the 7th week and the frequency of malformations in the child, even though the mother's blood glucose level is not the whole explanation.

At the diabetes centre at Rigshospitalet's Maternity Unit, we saw a significant fall in the number of congenital malformations from 7–8 % to 3–4 % in the beginning of the eighties [8]. The explanation of this favourable development was both that in the last part of the seventies, the diabetologists regulated especially the young diabetes patients much more strictly, and also that home monitoring had become more common, and haemoglobin A_{1c} was now being used clinically. In addition, a gynaecological clinic had been started in 1976 at Rigshospitalet for pre-conceptional guidance and planning of future pregnancy for referred diabetes patients. In the same clinic guidance was also given in safe contraception.

The Diabetes Centre at the Maternity Unit, Rigshospitalet (RH)

From the start of the Centre and until his death in 1978, Jørgen Pedersen (JP) had been responsible for the diabetological and partly also the organisational function at the Centre. After JP's death, the function as paid diabetes consultant was taken over by Claus Kühl (CK), who had already for several years been doing scientific work in the field of diabetes and pregnancy. When in 1988 CK had to give up his consultant function because of other work, the post was occupied by a temporary substitute, who stopped in 1990. At the same time, an appointment was made to a post as endocrinological consultant at RH, which the management thought could cover the function of diabetes consultant beside all other endocrinology including a consultant post that had just been abolished in the neurological department. Against this background, it was unrealistic that the diabetological function in the maternity ward could be carried out as hitherto. The function was undertaken by a succession of specialist registrars in the medical-nephrological department. Only in 2002, did the management realize that the situation was untenable. An endocrinological consultant with half of his job function in the maternity ward was appointed

It is a distinguishing feature of the Centre that so few different doctors and other staff have headed the work. In addition, the Centre has been favoured by having interested and able midwives and nurses from the very beginning. Among the changing specialist registrars, there has almost always been one with a particular interest in the specialty, and after 1978, a number of the research fellows attached to the Centre have participated in the clinical and scientific work.

Until 1978, the Centre had neither premises nor apparatus suited for research. In time as the scientific work became more and more laboratory-oriented, it was characteristic that the laboratory work took place elsewhere than at RH, for instance at Biochemical Institute, Steno Memorial Hospital, Sundby Hospital, Bispebjerg Hospital, and Danish Institute for Protein

Chemistry. This unsatisfying and untenable situation was changed in 1978, when research premises and offices, which still function satisfactorily today, were established in the south wing.

Another distinguishing feature of the Centre is that in the medical world it is better known abroad than in Denmark, and gradually as the number of publications in international journals grew in the 1960s, senior staff at the Centre were regularly invited as lecturers to various countries.

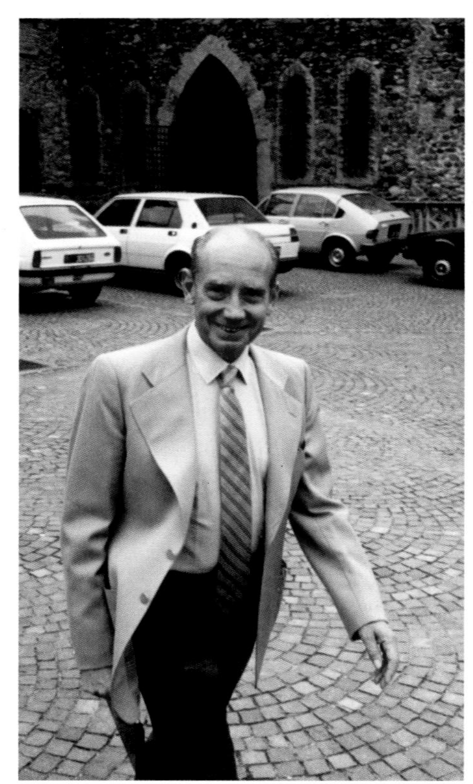

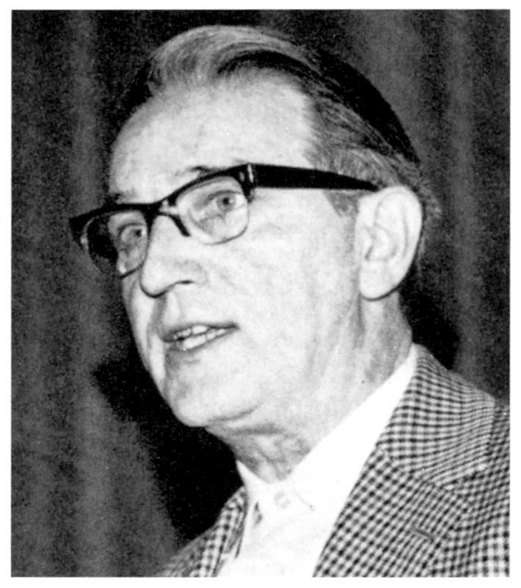

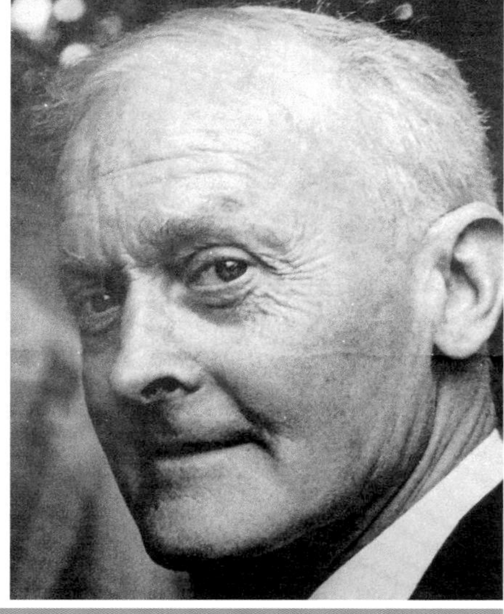

The Founding Fathers of the Diabetic Pregnancy Study Group (DPSG). From the left: Joseph Hoet, Jørgen Pedersen and John Stowers.

This has increased over the last twenty years so that the Centre's staff are now repeatedly invited each year to give lectures all around the world.

Another contributory factor to the positive global reputation of the Centre was the publication of Jørgen Pedersen's book in 1967 "*The pregnant diabetic and her newborn*", published in Polish in 1970 and with a radically revised edition in 1977, which also appeared in Spanish and Russian editions in 1979. The books are still frequently cited in articles on diabetes and pregnancy.

Diabetic Pregnancy Study Group (DPSG)

At the IDF (International Diabetes Federation) Congress in Stockholm in 1967, JP met two other European doctors, JJ Hoet, Belgium, and John Stowers, Scotland, who were both clinically and scientifically engaged in diabetes and pregnancy, The three colleagues formed a European "Diabetic Pregnancy Study Group" under EASD. In 1969, the group held its first half-day meeting in connection with EASD's annual meeting in Montpeiller, France. The three became the group's first "board members". The idea was to collect doctors who were working clinically and doing research in the field in an interdisciplinary group. This had 20 – now 35 – members. One can only be admitted to the group after endorsement by two members after having demonstrated one's scientific activity in the field. The following disciplines are represented: diabetology, obstetrics, paediatrics and what now goes under the designation of "basic science", comprising pathological anatomy, biochemistry and physiology. Guest speakers from widely different disciplines are invited to the annual working meetings.

The first meeting lasting more than one day was held in Denmark and arranged by JP in 1970. Since then, such working meetings have been held in various places, of which two more have been in Denmark. From 1977-80, I served as a board member, the last year as chairman. At the annual meetings since 1980, a JP memorial lecture has been given on a specialized topic and a JP medal has been awarded.

Five corresponding groups have been formed along the same lines: two in the USA, one in Australia/New Zealand, one in Japan and a quite new one in India. On this background, the *International Association of Diabetic Pregnancy Study Groups* (IADPSG) was founded in 1997 with two Danes being elected to the board, my replacement at RH, Peter Damm, and myself. The first meeting in IADPSG was held in Cairns, Australia in 1998, and the second meeting in 2003 in San Salvador, Comarruga, El Vendrell, Spain.

Type 2 diabetes and pregnancy

Our knowledge of the importance of pre-gestational diabetes (diabetes occurring before pregnancy) is preponderantly based on studies of women with type 1 diabetes. The reason for this is probably that type 2 diabetes in the childbearing age was formerly relatively rare, at least in Europe. Traditionally, pregnancy with type 2 diabetes was regarded as linked with considerably fewer problems than pregnancy with type 1 diabetes. There are, however, reports both from Denmark and from abroad that show that the number of pregnancies with type 2 diabetes is increasing [9]. At RH, the figure has risen from 6 per year in the period 1980-92 to 24 per year in the period 2002-05. There are a number of reasons for this. One of them is a changed population composition, in which a larger proportion of women in the childbearing age come from countries where the frequency of type 2 diabetes in younger adults is higher than in Denmark. Furthermore, we know that obesity/overweight and therefore probably also glucose intolerance/type 2 diabetes among younger women are rising. It must therefore be expected that the number of pregnancies with type 2 diabetes will continue to increase.

In the latest survey from RH from 1996-2001, 43 % of women with type 2 diabetes had a non-Caucasian background and less than 10 % of the pregnancies were planned. At the time of conception, 50 % were without treatment or treated with diet alone, while the rest were in tablet or insulin treatment. A total of 7.4 % were complicated with severe congenital malformations, and PM (perinatal mortality) was 7.4 %. In women with type 1 diabetes from the same period, the frequency of severe malformations was 3.9 % and PM 1.7 %.

These figures show that type 2 diabetes and pregnancy are in the situation that type 1 diabetes and pregnancy were in more than 20 years ago. Pregnancy and type 2 diabetes must therefore be taken seriously. An increased research effort in this field must therefore be regarded as necessary since it cannot be excluded that part of the morbidity in these pregnancies possibly may be due to components of the metabolic syndrome other than the metabolic regulation.

Early growth delay – ultrasound studies

In 1976, we began to carry out – a number of successive – ultrasound studies in the 1st trimester in all pregnant women with diabetes in order to determine the length of pregnancy. Quite surprisingly, we found that early in the diabetic pregnancy some foetuses were registered as smaller in the ultrasound measurements than expected from the calculation on the basis of the last menstruation. We used the term "early growth delay" [10]. There

was a significant link between early growth delay and the diabetes regulation, and correspondingly there has been a significant fall in the average growth delay over the last 20 years from 5.5 to 2.0 days, which must be ascribed to the effort to improve diabetes regulation around conception and in early pregnancy during the period concerned.

There was also found a significant link between early growth delay and the risk of congenital malformations. In the whole series of early ultrasound examinations of 376 children of mothers with type 1 diabetes, the chance of a good pregnancy outcome (defined as birth of a living, not malformed child) was lower in the group with growth delay, 85 % against 94 %, than in children with normal early growth. This highly significant difference shows that early growth delay is a real phenomenon and is not the result of uncertainty regarding the time of ovulation.

A group of children of mothers with diabetes was subsequently examined at the age of 4 and compared with a control group of children of non-diabetic mothers. All the children underwent the Denver Developmental Screening Test. In the control group, 88 % had a normal score in psychomotor development, while in the group with early growth delay only 69 % had a normal score. The children from the diabetes group without growth delay, on the other hand, scored exactly like the children in the control group. [11].

Gestational Diabetes Mellitus (GDM) = pregnancy diabetes

About 2 % of all pregnant women in Denmark develop GDM. The condition is defined as "carbon hydrate intolerance of varying severity diagnosed for the first time during pregnancy". The diagnosis is based on an oral glucose tolerance test (OGTT), and the condition is as a rule without symptoms. Pregnancy complicated by GDM is associated with increased maternal morbidity and perinatal mortality/morbidity. The risk of complications in the shorter or longer term can be reduced by diet treatment plus, possibly, insulin. Glucose tolerance is usually quickly normalised at the end of pregnancy, but the woman has a considerable risk of later developing type 2 diabetes. This has, for example, been shown in comprehensive follow-up studies from the Diabetes Center, RH [12]. In the most recent years, research at the Diabetes Centre has mainly been concerned with GDM. Four doctoral theses and three Ph.D. theses on the subject have been published.

Nationwide studies. Conclusion

The good results from the Diabetes Centre at RH, achieved since the mid-1980s, comprise, however, only about one-third of births with type 1 diabetes patients in Denmark. At RH's initiative a collaboration was started up in 1990 between the university hospitals in Copenhagen, Odense and Århus with Aalborg coming in later in order to obtain a nationwide overview of the outcomes of pregnancies in mothers with type 1 diabetes compared with the results from the background population. From 1993-99, all data on pregnancy, birth and the child for mothers with type 1 diabetes were registered prospectively in the Diabetes Association. In all 1,215 births – probably >90 % – were registered. The infant mortality was 3.1 % and the malformation frequency 5 %, where the corresponding figures for the population without diabetes were 0.75 % and 2.8 % respectively. Pregnancy toxaemia and premature birth were significantly higher for the diabetes patients. Only 34 % of the women had had daily monitoring of blood glucose around the time of conception, and 58 % had received pre-conceptional guidance [13].

Other nationwide studies from France and Holland also show frequencies for infant mortality and congenital malformations in diabetes pregnancies that are considerably higher than in the background population, and their results are not as good as those in Denmark.

In the St. Vincent Declaration in 1989, the goal was set that the results of diabetic pregnancies should approach the outcomes of non-diabetic pregnancies within 5 years. This goal has unfortunately not been attained.

Pregnancy in women with diabetes is still associated with considerably more complications surrounding pregnancy, birth and the post-natal period than in the background population. Especially women with poor diabetes regulation are in the highest risk group. Careful planning of the pregnancy with guided self-care based on daily blood monitoring of blood glucose before and during the pregnancy is an important step towards attaining the goal of the St. Vincent Declaration.

REFERENCES

1. *Brandstrup E, Okkels H. Pregnancy complicated with diabetes. Acta Obstet Gynecol Scand 1938;18:136-63*
2. *White P. Pregnancy complicating diabetes. Am J Med 1949;5:609-16*
3. *Mølsted-Pedersen L. Preterm labour and perinatal mortality in diabetic pregnancy-obstetric considerations. In: Sutherland HW, Stowers JM, eds. Carbohydrate metabolism in pregnancy and the newborn. Springer Verlag 1979:392-406*
4. *Pedersen J, Brandstrup E. Foetal mortality in pregnant diabetics. Lancet 1956;i: 607-10.*
5. *Mølsted-Pedersen L, Tygstrup I, Pedersen J. Congenital malformation in newborn infants of diabetic women. Lancet 1964;i:1964-8*
6. *Pedersen J, Mølsted-Pedersen L. Congenital malformations: The possible role of diabetes care outside pregnancy. In: Ciba Foundation Symposium 63. Pregnancy Metabolism, Diabetes and the fetus. Excerpta Medica 1979:265-71*
7. *Fuhrman K, Reiher H, Semmler V, Fischer F, Fischer M, Glockner E. Prevention of congenital malformations in infants of insulin-dependent diabetic mothers. Diabetes Care 1983;6:219-23*
8. *Damm P, Mølsted-Pedersen L. Significant decrease in congenital malformations in newborn infants of an unselected population of diabetic women. Am J Obstet Gynecol 1989;161:1163- 7*
9. *Clausen TD, Mathiesen E, Ekbom P, Hellmuth E, Mandrup-Poulsen T, Damm P. Poor pregnancy outcome in women with type 2 diabetes. Diab Care 2005;28:323-8*
10. *Pedersen JF, Mølsted-Pedersen L. Early growth retardation in diabetic pregnancy Br Med J 1979;1:18-9*
11. *Petersen MB, Pedersen SA, Greisen G, Pedersen JF, Mølsted-Pedersen L. Early growth delay in diabetic pregnancy: relation to psychomotor development age 4. Br Med J (Clin Res Ed) 1988;296:598-60*
12. *Lauenborg J, Hansen T, Jensen DM, Vestergaard H, Mølsted-Pedersen L, Hornnes, P, Locht H, Pedersen O, Damm P. Increasing incidence of diabetes after gestational diabetes – a long-term follow-up in a Danish population. Diabetes Care 2004;27:1194-9*
13. *Jensen DM, Damm P, Mølsted-Pedersen L, Ovesen P, Westergaard JG, Møller M, Beck-Nielsen H. Outcomes in Type 1 diabetic pregnancies. A nation-wide, population-based study. Diabetes Care 2004;27:2819-23*

EPIDEMIOLOGY, DATABASES AND BIOBANKS – A KEY TO INTERNATIONAL COOPERATION

KNUT BORCH-JOHNSEN

Epidemiology is the research discipline that concerns itself with the distribution of diseases in time and space and with the factors that underlie this distribution. The word epidemiology is formed from the two Greek words *epi* (on) and *demos* (people), and denotes research that is based on large groups of individuals, either by looking at large representative groups with a given disease (clinical epidemiology) or by sampling the total population (population-based epidemiology). Within the field of diabetes, epidemiologists work with such problems as the

- incidence of the disease in the population, regional and international variations in the incidence of the disease and the causes of this
- changes in the incidence of the disease over time and the causes of this
- prognosis of the disease (risk of complications developing or of mortality).

As epidemiologists typically concern themselves with large population groups – often with comparisons between countries – this is a research discipline that requires national and international cooperation among many groups. Epidemiological research has, however, had particularly favourable conditions in Denmark. Denmark has a number of national registers and databases, where both health data and social data are collected and stored from cradle to grave. Since 1967, we have had a personal identification number that accompanies each resident in Denmark throughout his or her life and can be used to collect data on many people from many sources by linking the registers using the personal identification number as a key. Only very few countries have this possibility, which is an important precondition for the strong international position held by Danish epidemiology within both types of diabetes as well as a large number of other diseases. In the course of the most recent decades, a number of large national biobanks containing blood samples, urine samples, genetic material and other biological material have been established. These biobanks have further extended the possibilities for epidemiological research and have strengthened the cooperation between epidemiologists and researchers in a number of other disciplines.

Epidemiology and prevention in the light of history

Epidemiology is classically divided into descriptive epidemiology, which is concerned with who and how many incur the disease, with the prognosis of the disease and possibly also with its societal and economic consequences, while analytic (cause-seeking) epidemiology is the name given to the epidemiological studies whose purpose it is to identify causes of the disease (circumstances that are accompanied by an increased or reduced risk for development of the disease) and to identify factors that affect the prognosis once the disease has developed.

Even though epidemiology did not break through in earnest as a scientific method until around the 1950s, it is far from being a new discipline. Several major advances of importance for disease prevention occurred in the 1850s. The best known example dates from the mid-1850s, when cholera caused a disturbingly high mortality not least among children in some parts of London, while in adjacent areas of the town there was markedly lower morbidity and mortality. In 1855 by systematically mapping incidences of the disease and the water supplies to the individual households, Doctor John Snow was able to link a number of occurrences of the disease to a certain water pump, "the Broad Street Pump". By further collating information about water pipes with sewage pipes, it could be shown that the reason why this particular pump caused cholera was that leaky water and sewage pipes were placed so close to one another that the drinking water was polluted. Prevention therefore consisted of renovating the water and sewage pipes, and with knowledge of when and where the disease had spread, prevention was possible even without knowing the real cause: the bacterium Vibrio cholerae.

Diabetes epidemiology – in Denmark

At one blow, the discovery of insulin in 1921 made it possible for patients to survive for many decades. However, the problem was not solved, since the possibility of treating diabetes unmasked the link between diabetes and the risk of developing complications in the eyes, kidneys, nerve paths and blood circulation. Naturally, this observation raised the question – "why?" – and the answer to it could be provided only through cooperation between a large number of research disciplines comprising, for instance, clinical research, physiology, epidemiology, genetics and molecular biology. With the possibility of treatment, the question of the disease's incidence also became relevant, and the need to study the occurrence of the different types of diabetes arose in various parts of the world.

Complications and prognosis – it begins in Århus

The elucidation of the epidemiology of the diabetes complications and their causal factors is a field in which the Danish research tradition is both long and strong. With his base in the University of Aarhus, Knud Lundbæk carried out comprehensive studies of the late-diabetic complications, and in 1953 on the basis of his research, it was possible to classify the complications in groups that both had common features and also behaved in such a way that Lundbæk divided them into microvascular complications (complications linked to small blood vessels, comprising eyes, kidneys, nerve paths) and macrovascular complications (primarily comprising the changes associated with arteriosclerosis in the large and medium-size blood vessels, changes that lead to heart disease, cerebral haemorrhage/blood clots in the brain and to reduced blood supply, especially to the feet and the lower extremities). This classification has held since 1953 and is still used to classify the late-diabetic complications.

The story from Gentofte

In order to elucidate the prognosis of type 1 diabetes in particular, the first classical cohort studies on Danish patients were carried out at the then Steno Memorial Hospital. Under the leadership of Torsten Deckert, the study followed up on how all the patients with type 1 diabetes who had been referred to the hospital and who had developed diabetes before 1952 had fared. By comparing the patients who incurred diabetes in the 1920s and 1930s with those who did so in the 1940s and 1950s, it could be shown that the survival rate rose markedly over this period and markedly more than would have been expected on the basis of the general development in morbidity and mortality in Denmark. The studies also showed that patients who went to regular check-ups fared better than those who did not.

Finally, the studies indicated that even in a small country like Denmark, there was regional variation in the risk of developing severe complications and of dying of diabetes. Especially this last conclusion was both medi-

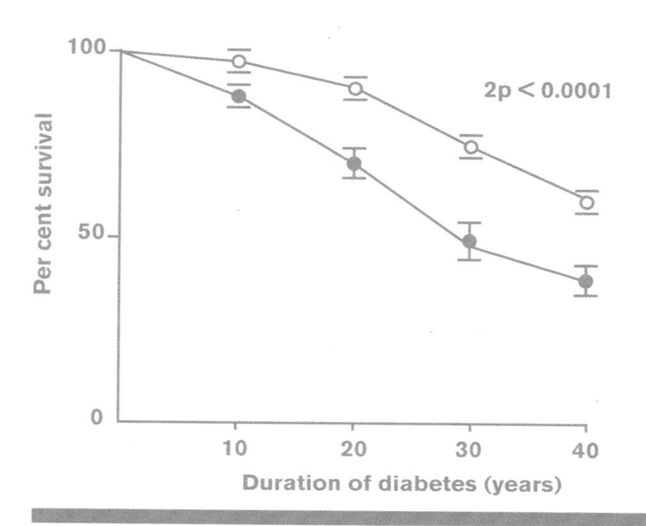

Regular control of diabetes helps. The figure shows survival in patients with type 1 diabetes. All patients were admitted to Steno Memorial Hospital for regulation and instruction in diabetes care within the first five years of the disease. Attenders *continued to attend regular check-up at Steno Memorial Hospital,* Non-attenders *sought other pastures. (Data from Torsten Deckert).*

cally and politically controversial and therefore met considerable resistance in Danish medical circles. In the course of the 1980s, Deckert's colleagues under his guidance conducted a series of further studies on the prognosis of type 1 diabetes. In this way, the importance of diabetic kidney disease as a risk factor for

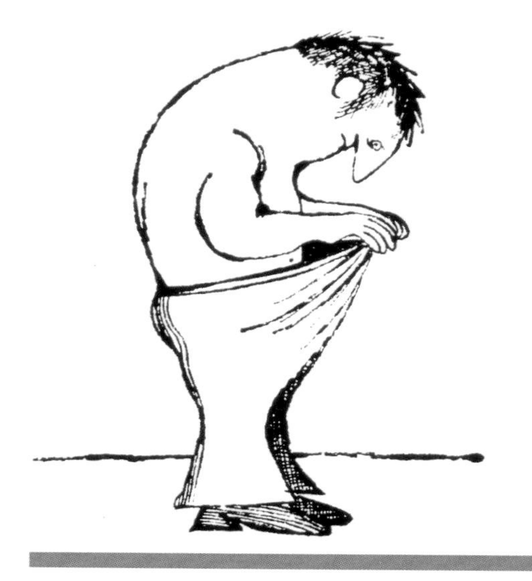

Is there albuminuria?

dying not only of renal failure, but even more so of cardiovascular disease became evident, and it also became clear that there was a very close link between the severe stages of microvascular (small blood vessel) and macrovascular (large blood vessel) complications. Thus, diabetes patients could develop mild degrees of changes in the nerve paths and in the blood vessels of the eye, but the patients who developed more severe eye changes with newly formed blood vessels, called proliferative retinopathy, and patients who developed diabetic renal disease characterized by increased secretion of protein in the urine were those who died early and indeed often of cardiovascular disease. Together with the findings of a number of clinical and experimental studies, this gave rise to the research group putting forward the so-called "Steno hypothesis", in which it was proposed that albuminuria is a marker of the presence of a generalized blood vessel dysfunction, for which reason two new concepts were introduced: benign and malign diabetic angiopathy (disease of the blood vessels), in which it is the latter that progresses fastest and binds the micro- and macrovascular vessel changes together

The hypothesis also offered a possible explanation of the underlying mechanisms and physiological differences between individuals that could lead to the fact that some people develop benign and others malign angiopathy. While the latter part is still the subject of scientific discussion, the first part is now a well-established fact for patients with both type 1 and type 2 diabetes. It has subsequently been shown in both Danish and foreign studies that even relatively mild albuminuria is a marker of generalized blood vessel disorder, surprisingly so also in individuals without diabetes. These studies had great importance for the prioritization of the focus of the subsequent clinical work, and as recently as in 2007, the Danish National Board of Health's recommendations as to how the treatment of patients with diabetes should best be undertaken (the Process Programme for Chronic Disease) pointed out that patients with very slightly increased secretion of albumin in the urine (microalbuminuria) constitute a special risk group, for which the treatment poses very special requirements and should therefore be centralized to a certain extent.

At the same time the studies had a purely practical effect for patients with diabetes. The demonstration that the patients with type 1 diabetes who do not develop diabetic renal disease can expect to live almost as long as persons without diabetes (on average 5 to 7 years shorter) brought about considerable relaxations concerning access to take out life and accident insurance and also led to considerably better access to adoption for this large group of patients.

An old wives' tale from the 1980s

An odd story from Gentofte, which is still the object of international research activity, was the demonstration in 1984 of a possible link between the duration of the breastfeeding period and the child's risk of developing type 1 diabetes. The starting point was a Canadian study of a special strain of rats with a particularly high risk of developing diabetes, in which the researchers could show both that the composition of the diet was of great importance for whether the animals developed diabetes, and also that breastfeeding appears to protect newborn infants against a number of infections inasmuch as the mother's milk directly protects the newborn infant. Against this background, Jørn Nerup and Knut Borch-Johnsen raised the question: "Can nutrition in early infancy affect the risk of type 1 diabetes, and does breast milk contain protective factors?". By comparing the development and duration of breastfeeding and the incidence of type 1 diabetes in the Scandinavian countries, it could be shown that at the same time as breastfeeding frequency fell, the incidence of diabetes rose. After this, the breastfeeding pattern in families with more than one child, at least one of whom had diabetes, was examined. On average, children who developed diabetes were breastfed for a shorter time than their healthy siblings, and a number of them had never been breastfed. With this, the conclusion was in the bag, and the article was submitted. The critical editor was naturally sceptical and rejected the findings as improbable. A new group of diabetes children was traced, and the result was the same. The article was sent off to the same journal, the same editor, with the words: "We understand your healthy scepticism. However, we have repeated the study and confirmed our findings – do you dare now?" The article was printed and a number of similar studies followed, but now, 20 years later, it is still not entirely clear whether this was a true observation or just an old wives' tale from Gentofte.

The incidence of diabetes – the major population studies

During the 1970s, the first systematic studies were carried out in Denmark of how many persons under 30 years of age develop type 1 diabetes. The work was based on two centres, one in Odense with Anders Green as the driving force and the other at Steno Memorial Hospital under Jørn Nerup. In this way, it was determined not only that Denmark is among the countries that has the highest incidence of type 1 diabetes, but that regional differences in the incidence of diabetes could also be demonstrated. Both on Funen and in Gentofte the work continued on elucidating the incidence and possible causes of type 1 diabetes in children and young people in Denmark. Thus, the first demonstration that nutrition in earliest infancy has an effect on the risk of developing type 1 diabetes is a Danish observation, which has subsequently led to wide-scale research nationally and internationally.

It was however not until the establishment of the nationwide register comprising all who develop diabetes before the age of 16 that the overall picture of the incidence of diabetes in Denmark was obtained. The register will be described later in this chapter.

As for the incidence of type 2 diabetes, this was systematically described for the first time in Denmark as part of the so-called "Population Studies" in Glostrup. The initiative for these studies was taken by Per From Hansen, who on a visit to the USA was inspired by the Framingham Study. However, it was by no means easy to carry out these studies in Denmark. It was difficult to find support for the idea that healthy, well-functioning persons could teach us anything about the causes of disease. For example, when From Hansen presented the idea of population studies at a meeting of consultants at Glostrup Hospital, he was met with headshaking disapproval, while some colleagues openly stated that it was not just a waste of money, but "crystal-clear madness". For the population studies in Glostrup, certain birth cohorts in selected municipalities around Glostrup County Hospital were invited to a comprehensive health check, which included a check as to whether they had diabetes.

Over the last 50 years, studies of the population in and around Glostrup have been carried out. The activities now take place at the Research Centre for Prevention and Health, but these studies have contributed to creating a precise picture of the very rapid rise in the incidence of type 2 diabetes in Denmark over the last 30 years. Under the leadership of Knut Borch-Johnsen, first as head of the Centre in Glostrup, later at Steno Diabetes Center, it has been shown that the incidence of diabetes from 1974 to 1996 rose by more than 50 %, and that the increase has further continued up to today (2005). The increase can essentially be explained by the fact that on average we weigh more and are less physically active than formerly. These two circumstances are fully sufficient to explain the development.

Causes of diabetes – an epidemiological challenge

An understanding of a disease's causes is as already mentioned not necessarily an absolute precondition for prevention, but, all things being equal, it makes things easier. It was, however, not primarily diabetes that was in mind when Tage Kemp, Mogens Hauge and Bent Harvald established the Twin Registry in 1954. Their goal was to use studies of one-egg and two-egg twins to study the effect of chronic diseases. One-egg twins share inherited material and environment, whereas two-egg twins are genetically just as different as other siblings, apart from sharing the same environment both in the womb and in childhood. This register has been crucial for a number of important findings in the field of diabetes.

It has been shown by Flemming Pociot on the basis of this register that the inheritability of type 1 diabetes is higher than had been expected on the basis of ordinary family studies, but perhaps even more convincingly the Twin Register has contributed to the understanding of the inheritability of type 2 diabetes. Inheritability (understood as the risk that twin 2 of one-egg twins will get the disease if twin 1 has developed it) is higher for type 2 than for type 1 diabetes, as shown by Allan Vaag's research group. This is the case despite the fact that the hereditary succession is probably far more complex in type 2 diabetes. The same group has also used twin studies to investigate the importance of life in the womb for later risk of disease. It has been convincingly documented that low birth weight and therewith poor life conditions in the womb have an effect on the individual's insulin sensitivity and risk of getting diabetes decades later. Again this is an example of the fact that the establishment of registers and databases has acquired an importance that was absolutely impossible to imagine when the three pioneers laid the foundation for the Twin Register.

The Inuit population in Greenland – a special challenge

Further north – in Greenland – studies by Sagild from 1962 indicated that diabetes was largely non-existent among the Inuit. The method of investigation he used was not optimal, but with it he found a diabetes incidence

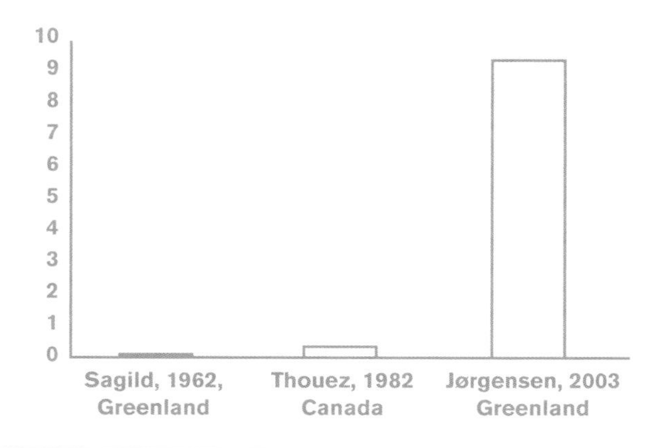

Diabetes prevalence among Inuit in Greenland and Canada. (Data from the author).

of 6 per 10,000 corresponding to 25–35 cases in all Greenland. Systematic population studies in 1999 in both Nuuk and in a number of small towns and settlements showed that the incidence in the adult population has now risen to about 1 per 10 inhabitants or between 2,500 and 3,500 occurrences in all Greenland.

In this way, the Inuit of Greenland joined the ever-growing list of large and small people's all over the world, who in step with a shift towards the European or North-American lifestyle have become very vulnerable to sudden changes in their living conditions.

Diabetes epidemiology in an international perspective

Diabetes was one of the first fields in which an international network was established with a view to epidemiological research. There are many explanations for this, and it was the product of the interaction between clear, unsolved scientific problems, powerful personalities and very special political conditions in Europe. The scientific problem was the late-diabetic complications, about which certain circles held that there were regional and international variations in the risk of developing complications. If this presumption could be confirmed, it would also create the basis for models explaining the causes of these differences. The powerful personalities were a generation of diabetes researchers with a strong scientific and international commitment, who came from such countries as England, France, Switzerland and the DDR and all combined their clinical work and experimental research with an interest in epidemiology. The political scene was a Europe split between East and West, in which the Berlin Wall from 1961 was yet another example of how the populations in the two parts of Europe were separated. There was a great wish to create a basis for the free exchange of knowledge across borders. This cocktail of three ingredients led both to the carrying out of the first WHO study of diabetes and also to the formation of the scientific association European Diabetes Epidemiology Group (EDEG), which became the first of a now large number of specialist associations in European diabetes research. The WHO study in 1967 was planned with the object of studying regional and international variation in the development of late-diabetic complications.

Subsequently, initiatives have been taken via the same group for a series of studies. In 1986, the group was the base for the planning of the EU-supported project – EURODIAB, whose Danish arm was undertaken by, among others, Anders Green from Odense. The study had three arms, but especially in the field of type 1 diabetes, it achieved ground-breaking results through the mapping of regional variation and by identifying special areas in Sardinia and Finland where the incidence was particularly high.

At the same time, this cooperation created the foundation for international cooperation among geneticists, epidemiologists, immunologists and clinicians in the further identification of genetic and environmental risk factors for development of both type 1 and type 2 diabetes.

The big databases and international cooperation

EDEG was also the starting point for the establishment of the so-called DECODE study. This study assembled knowledge from a large number of studies with the originally collected data of almost 30 population studies being given entirely free of charge to a single large database placed under Jaakko Tuomilehto in Helsingfors. By thus collecting these data in one large database comprising more than 50,000 individuals, it became possible to generate entirely new knowledge about the determinants of morbidity and mortality for type 2 diabetes. The study was inspired by a proposal from the American Diabetes Association that the diagnostic criteria for diabetes should be changed. The study documented the undesirability of abandoning the present criteria for the diagnosis, but the knowledge that the study generated helped to place focus on the importance of the blood glucose levels of non-fasting patients for the development of cardiovascular disease in particular.

The role of the biobanks in epidemiological research

In step with the movement from descriptive to analytic epidemiology, the use of biological markers from blood specimens, urine specimens, etc. has become an ever-more important part of the research. In recent years, advances in the field of genetics have provided further possibilities of identifying individuals with an especially high risk of developing diabetes or the accompanying complications. By not merely taking blood specimens and analysing them, but by also preserving them for decades, it has proved possible to exploit the major population studies even more effectively. In this way material from biobanks has helped to elucidate the quantitative importance of, for example, microalbuminuria, homocystein, Nt-pro-BNP and a number of inflammation markers for the risk of developing cardiovascular disease.

The biobanks are also absolutely vital for the major international cooperative projects involving geneticists/molecular biologists and epidemiologists in elucidating the interaction between genes and environment in relation to the risk of developing, for example, diabetes. These studies require such a large patient material that it is unrealistic to imagine that individual groups can perform the studies alone. The establishment of biobanks is an investment in the future just as the major epidemiological studies that have been conducted in Denmark. From the establishment of the major population studies in Glostrup and Østerbro, between 10 and 20 years passed before they became scientifically active in earnest. In contrast, they now constitute invaluable databases for research. The same applies to biobanks. They collect data on large population groups, but they only become interesting when something happens to the persons who are registered. On the other hand, they contain in various contexts biological material that is just waiting to be used for research.

The blood specimen cards from Danish infants, who are systematically examined for phenylketonuria, are an example of such material, which is now proving useful in many other contexts.

A task that should be taken up by the Danish research environment is to systematize the information on what biobanks there are in order to ensure that the material the population has made available to researchers is in fact used optimally. Correspondingly, it is incumbent on legislators to ensure that the rights and integrity of the citizens are protected and that society and its citizens at the same time can be sure that the many data and information that have been registered can also be used for research that will benefit the individual and society as a whole. This requires a careful ethical balancing of the various concerns to avoid a situation in which both too high a degree of liberalism and too high a degree of restrictiveness will have a destructive effect on epidemiological research and the prevention of disease.

Diabetes epidemiology – quo vadis?

The epidemiological studies in the field of diabetes have given a clear picture of the global problem we are facing in respect of both type 1 and type 2 diabetes. They have also contributed to our understanding of why the incidence of diabetes is rising worldwide and thereby of where the preventive focus should be concentrated. Furthermore, the studies have contributed to the identification of both genetic and other biological markers for diabetes. However, this does not change the fact that we are facing great challenges that will continue to inspire epidemiologists and other researchers in Denmark and the rest of the world.

It is now 86 years since it became possible to treat diabetes with insulin. It is more than 30 years since the HLA system's importance for the risk of developing type 1 diabetes became known, but despite this, we know very little about why only some of those individuals who are genetically disposed to do so develop diabetes. Identification of the risk factors that trigger such a development is a typical epidemiological task, but to date, there have been only small and limited successes. Here we have one of the most essential challenges. For both type 1 diabetes and type 2 diabetes, by far the greater part of the scientific literature is based on European and North-American studies and thereby on an ethnic group that constitutes only a small part of the world's population.

Epidemiological and physiological studies increasingly show that risk factors for the development of diabetes and diabetes-related complications manifest their effects very differently in different ethnic groups. In other words, we cannot uncritically transfer knowledge about the causes of the disease from one population group to another. There is therefore a need for the epidemiological studies to be moved out into those parts of the world that will first and foremost produce the largest growth in the number of diabetes patients in coming decades in Asia, Africa and South America.

Epidemiology has been more successful in the field of type 2 diabetes with regard to identifying important risk factors. One limitation here is that we tend to perceive type 2 diabetes as one disease despite the fact that the course of the disease, the needed treatment and the link to classical risk factors such as obesity and physical activity exhibit a very considerable degree of heterogeneity. If our understanding of the causes of the disease is to become better, it will be necessary that future studies can to a far higher degree identify the individual sub-groups that together constitute type 2 diabetes. Here epidemiology plays a role in the characterization and identification of the relevant, highly selected sub-groups. This strategy requires a change of mentality both in the epidemiological and the molecular-biological research environments. For many years, the philosophy has been that "big is beautiful". In the future, we shall still need comprehensive studies in order to find the special sub-groups, but the real scientific focus should subsequently be on extremely well characterized sub-groups, in which clinically significant differences can be seen even in small populations.

CLINICAL TRIALS FOR EVIDENCE-BASED CLINICAL PRACTICE

BO FELDT-RASMUSSEN

Introduction

Evidence-based medicine (EBM) is about documentation of the effects and side effects of drugs and other forms of treatment. The documentation is best when it is based on well planned, well designed, and often very large and costly clinical trials. The health services of today cannot exist without EBM – a concept that has become a mantra over the past 20 years. Without EBM, it is not possible to draw up guidelines for the clinical treatment of diseases, including of course diabetes. My good friend Professor Andrew Boulton from Manchester, UK, has a slide he often shows in his clinical lectures. The text spells out the status of EBM today: "*In God we trust – all others have to provide evidence*".

The medical world has not always been equally aware of the importance of documented knowledge rather than faith and experience. And, indeed, in some cases it may seem unnecessary. The use of insulin to save the lives of patients with type 1 diabetes has for instance never been tested in a scientifically structured clinical trial. Only a short time passed after the first injections of insulin in Toronto in 1922, before the necessity of introducing systematic insulin treatment of all type 1 diabetes patients was recognized. One couldn't wait for the clinically controlled trials because insulin simply worked. Before the fantastic days in Toronto, the patients died – after the discovery they lived. In most cases, however, it is obvious that today we must and should base our treatment strategies and guidelines on EBM and thereby on studies that follow the rules for Good Clinical Practice (GCP).

A good example is the "Heart Protection Study". This study documented the effects of cholesterol-lowering treatment using the preparation *Simvastatin®*. The evidence was moved from belief to knowledge. The treatment improved survival chances for large groups of patients, and the effect was best among patients with diabetes. The Danish Health Service's subsidy rules for cholesterol-lowering treatment were liberalized a few weeks after publication of these results. The need for EBM is also seen in the innumerable examples that show that recommendation of treatments without documented effect can give patients exaggerated hopes, unnecessary inconvenience and large but fruitless expense. One instance is counselling for weight-reducing diet treatment and other treatment of overweight type 2 diabetes patients. Here, over the years, the recommendations for the distribution of the diet have ranged from high consumption of carbohydrates, via high consumption of protein to high consumption of fat, possibly accompanied by undocumented expensive dietary supplements! Unfortunately, this would also appear to describe the state of things in the year 2007. Finally, the use of EBM can also do something about the problem that the undocumented treatments that are introduced may not merely be without effect, but may be also directly dangerous for patients.

A little about EBM and guidelines

The scale that is used to assess the documentation available ranges from level 1, which is the highest and best level, to level 4. The lowest level, level 4, requires that at least one person (a physician), who treats patients, has experience of the effect of a given treatment: "It is my experience that...." The best level, level 1, requires that there are results from a number of correctly performed studies, and that these results are subjected to a systematic review – a meta-analysis – which with certainty documents a clinically significant effect. Thus, there must be more than one single correctly performed study that shows an effect. Level 2 concerns evidence obtained in a single correctly performed clinical trial, and at level 3, one finds a broad array of more modest requirements of the quality of the studies. It is my assessment, that the first 50 years of the 75-year period we are concerned with here were dominated by treatments with documentation at evidence levels 3 to 4. Didn't the treatments work then? No doubt they did in most cases, and this should make the reader realize that a treatment may well be effective without being documented in accordance with modern requirements. The explanation why the requirements of documentation are today at levels 1-2 should, among other things, be seen in the light of the fact that many new treatments are very expensive in comparison with the classical forms of treatment they are designed to replace. The principles of EBM are used in order to reach a decision as to whether they are better, and whether they are worth the extra expense.

A little about evidence-based medicine and about diabetes 30 years ago

I studied medicine at the University of Copenhagen in the period 1971 to 1978. Also at that time there were many deeply committed persons in the medical world. Among these were Professor Henrik R. Wulff and consultant Bjørn Andersen, who had assumed the great task of teaching students and the rest of the medical world about the clinically controlled trial and its importance. Through the textbook "Rational Diagnosis and Treatment" (Oxford: Blackwell 1976, 1981 and 2000), we were introduced to the sins of the past, which had led to many unnecessary treatments, and we learnt about the advantages of the clinically controlled trial. In 1978, when I had just taken my finals, diabetes was the most frequent cause of acquired blindness. Diabetic nephropathy was a complication that developed in almost half of all type 1 diabetes patients. Once the kidney disease had developed, the survival term was only about 7 years. The offer of dialysis for these unfortunate patients had not yet materialized in earnest. Dying younger patients were often admitted to Steno Memorial Hospital. They died of kidney failure.

The importance of glycaemic regulation was a topic that was subject to lively debate. There was no convincing documentation that it meant anything at all. A couple of years earlier, my mentor Torsten Deckert had for example written an article entitled "*Diabetic nephropathy – fault or destiny?*" According to this work, it was not possible to demonstrate that good regulation of diabetes had any effect on the development of diabetic renal disease. Torsten Deckert and his mentor Jakob E Poulsen concluded cautiously: "*We do not believe that diabetic control is* irrelevant *to the development of nephropathy, but destiny rather than faults in treatment seem to be of importance in the development of nephropathy in insulin-dependent diabetes*". There was something to it, but with the knowledge we have today, Torsten Deckert would probably change the order of the factors, placing good regulation before destiny. It is a good thing for the patient that this is the way it is, because we can do something about regulation.

The importance of blood pressure lowering treatment had not been finally documented either. Progress was being made in that direction, as also with the documentation of the effect of laser treatment of proliferative retinopathy (severe changes in the eyes with newly formed blood vessels). In the next 10 to 15 years evidence-based knowledge was generated about all these factors: glycaemic regulation, blood pressure reduction, laser treatment, cholesterol-lowering treatment, and lifestyle changes. A large part of the documentation came from studies from Danish and other Nordic research groups. In the following, I shall describe how I observed and participated in this work, and I shall focus on the fields in which I was most involved or where I was very close to events. I shall therefore devote particular attention to describing how the effect of good diabetes regulation and of blood pressure lowering treatment was documented.

Steno Memorial Hospital – a unique place to be for a young researcher

I was employed at Steno Memorial Hospital (SMH) in 1983. During the first week, I had talks about my research possibilities with all three editors of this book. They were at that time *the consultants* at SMH. This led to what has so far been 25 years of research into diabetic nephropathy and cardiovascular diseases with constant support and stimulation from my mentor and friend Torsten Deckert. In the course of a short time, I had met colleagues at SMH and from other centres who were already or would later become prominent figures in research and other developments in the Danish and international health systems. In a few days, I had met not only Torsten Deckert, Christian Binder and Jørn Nerup but also Hans-Henrik Parving, Jens Sandahl Christiansen, Torsten Lauritzen (Little Torsten), Knut Borch-Johnsen, Thomas Mandrup-Poulsen, Birger Thorsteinsson,

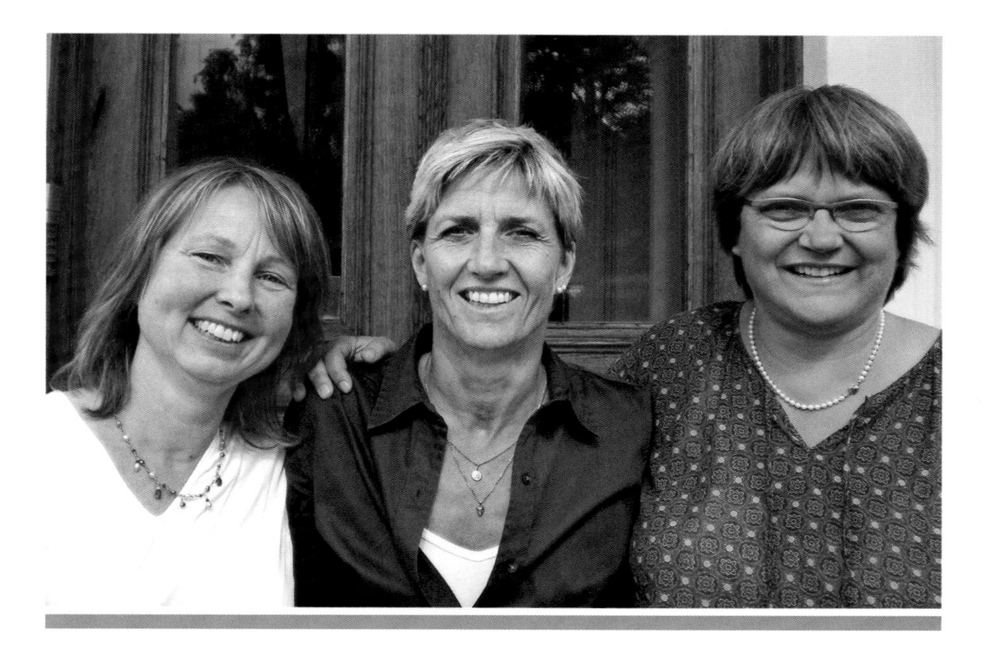

The Parving Sisters. Three important women in Hans-Henrik Parving's research group. From the left: Eva Hommel, Mari-Anne Gall and Elisabeth Mathiesen.

Stig Pramming and Svend Hartling. There were not enough office facilities, so Birger and I shared an office in a temporary wooden building erected for the purpose in the grounds of SMH. We called it "Domus Vakkelvorn [= ramshackle]", inspired by the name given to the villa of the founder of SMH: "Domus Hagedorn".

Later came "the Parving Sisters": Elisabeth Mathiesen, Mari-Anne Gall and Eva Hommel. I am still in contact and work together with them all at various levels. Within six months, I had met many of the big Danish names outside SMH: Carl Erik Mogensen, Henning Beck-Nielsen, Oluf Pedersen, Jannik Hilsted, Sten Madsbad, and then there's not space to mention all those who were there already or who arrived later.

For my own field of research, it was not long before Torsten, my mentor, had introduced me to all internationally important colleagues: Harry Keen, GianCarlo Viberti, Kristian Hanssen, Michael Mauer, Michael Steffes and many, many more. Torsten's technique was sublime. He would introduce me to a big gun and start up a conversation. The first time the "gun" addressed me, Torsten would slip away, so the "gun" was stuck in a discussion with me, and a new part of my network was established.

As a rule, we had access to relatively generous funding, but there were also periods when Christian Binder, who had the administrative responsibility, demanded restraint. Christian introduced something as unheard of as a research budget, which had to be adhered to. This was a peep into the future, and certainly not something we were used to. In one such period, Torsten asked me to buy isotopes, insulin pumps and a fitness cycle for our projects. I remember being worried. Hadn't Christian just said that we were out of funds? But I remember Torsten's unconcerned style: "*It's all right for you to order them. You understand, Christian is a little ambivalent in his relation to money. Sometimes we have to save and sometimes we can buy. Now we're buying!*"

That drive and of course also Christian's administrative responsibility were the fuel that obtained the economic means necessary to plan and carry out the so-called Steno Studies, which helped to prove the value of good diabetes regulation.

The importance of glycaemic control

As already mentioned, the importance of blood glucose regulation was unclarified for the major part of the 75 years. *Diabetic nephropathy – fault or destiny?* It was necessary to wait for good and not all too expensive methods for home monitoring of blood glucose. It was also necessary to wait for measurements of HbA_{1c}, which gives the blood glucose level over longer periods. Finally, it was necessary to wait for effective methods of improving the blood glucose regulation over a longer period. This was a matter of, for instance, pump treatment and treatment with many daily insulin injections. With the development of these methods and techniques, it became possible to perform so-called prospective, randomized studies of standard-glycaemic versus improved-glycaemic regulation. Then followed a number of studies all around the world.

The most well known, from the beginning of the 1980s, came from the USA (Kroc), Denmark and Norway (The Oslo Study). Among the most famous are two insulin pump studies from SMH. The first Steno Study was planned and headed by Torsten Deckert and research fellow Torsten Lauritzen. I myself was responsible for the second Steno Study together with research fellow Elisabeth Mathiesen. With the Steno Studies, Torsten had insisted that SMH could do that kind of thing itself. There was no reason to drown oneself in large multi-centre studies like the American Kroc studies and later the Diabetes Control and Complication Trial (DCCT). Strong forces were working against the local SMH concept, but Torsten's insistence led to the fundamental knowledge concerning the favourable effect of near-normal blood glucose regulation being produced in Denmark, Norway and Sweden. It was not until many years later that that effect was confirmed and raised to evidence level 1 by the DCCT study.

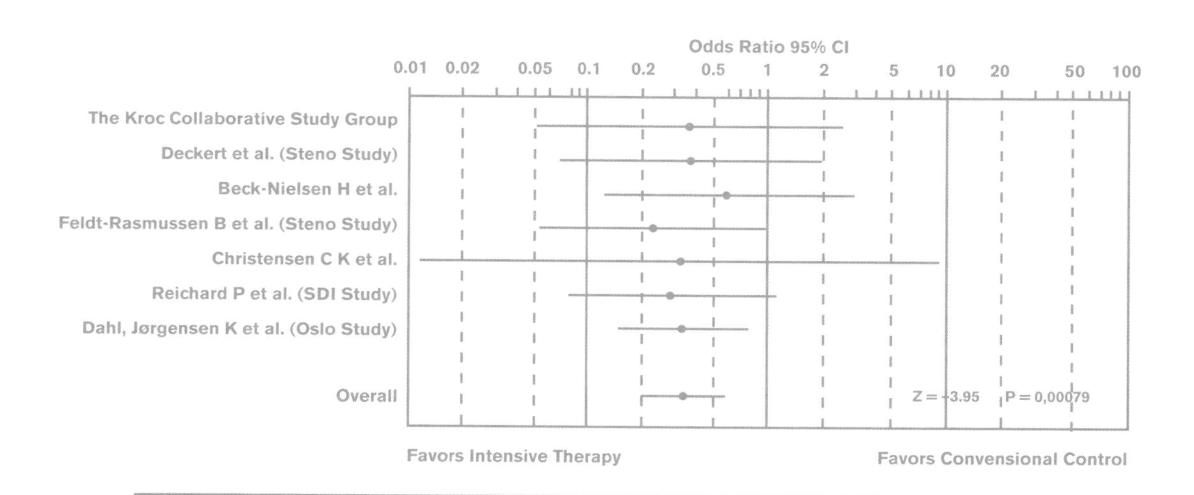

Effect of intensive blood glucose control on the progression of diabetic renal disease. Data before the results of the DCCT Study arrived in 1993. (Wang et al, Lancet 1993).

In the second Steno Insulin Pump Study, we treated and followed a total of 36 patients, 18 of whom were treated with insulin pump. We ourselves, Marja Deckert and Hanne Foght, who were technicians on the project, knew the patients and their closest families at an almost personal level. The GCP rules had not been invented. We ourselves made the envelopes that were used for randomization of the patients. We had ourselves gone around with the pumps, though with salt water instead of insulin. We knew from our own experience most of the problems that the pumps could cause before we instructed the patients. All the patients were given our private telephone numbers, and they used them. We were glad together with our patients when after one year's treatment the study showed that we had stopped the development of the preliminary stage of diabetic renal disease.

The sum of the observations from these minor "pre-DCCT" studies all indicated that it was important to improve the glycaemic regulation. A

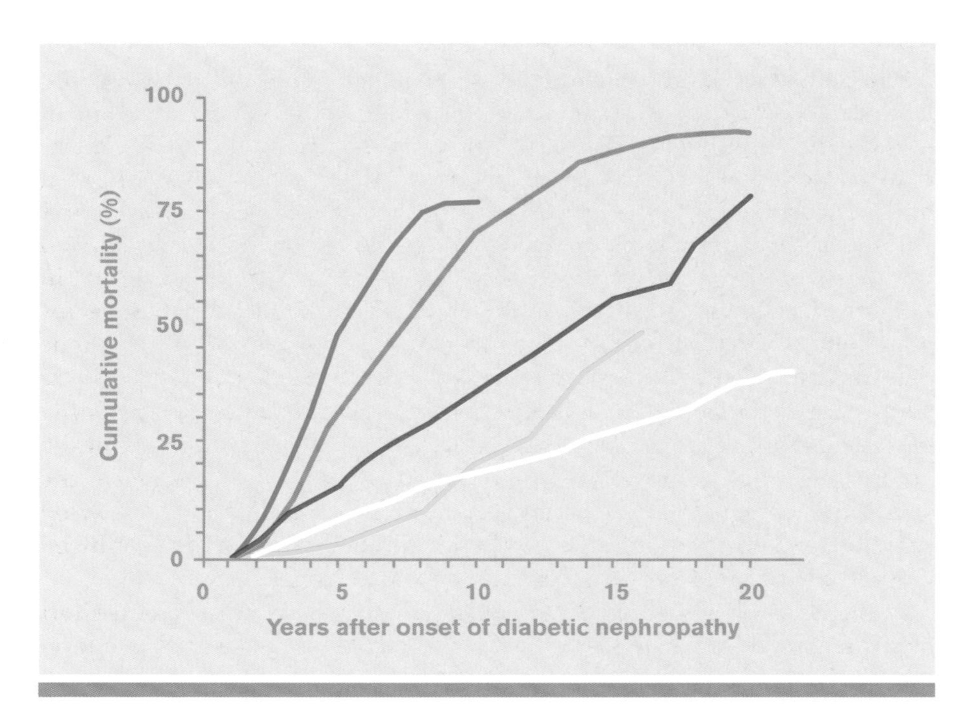

The cumulative mortality after onset of renal disease could be reduced from 75 % to 15 % over 25 years.
Blue: Knowles 1971; green: Andersen 1983; yellow: Parving 1996; red: Rossing 1996; white: Astrup 2005. (Kidney International, 2006).

meta-analysis of the 7 best studies concluded in 1993: "*Long-term intensive regulation of blood glucose reduces the risk of diabetic retinopathy and the progression of nephropathy, but in insulin pump treatment there is an increased risk of hypoglycaemia and ketoacidosis*". We thus got past the meta-analysis's evidence levels 1–2 before the publication of the American DCCT. The DCCT swept away the last doubts. For patients with type 2 diabetes the United Kingdom Prospective Diabetes Study (UKPDS) delivered corresponding evidence of the importance of glycaemic regulation. Today, all guidelines recommend that the glycaemic regulation should be optimized in accordance with defined treatment goals. The evidence level is 1.

We no longer believe. We know.

Blood pressure lowering treatment in connection with diabetic nephropathy

A couple of Danish groups must be mentioned among the pioneers who helped to show how important raised blood pressure is for the development of diabetic renal disease. One of the groups was headed by the newly appointed Professor Carl Erik Mogensen from Århus, and the other was led by the young specialist registrar from Steno Memorial Hospital Hans Henrik Parving. At the same time, corresponding studies were being conducted in other countries. One of the major groups was from Guy's Hospital in London. The design of the studies was by and large identical. Small groups of patients with positive urine strips for protein, so-called clinical diabetic nephropathy, were followed for a couple of years with their blood pressure being observed and without anything special being done about the glycaemic regulation. That was the treatment level of the day, so it was ethically acceptable. After this period of observation, treatment was begun – the so-called "Early aggressive antihypertensive treatment". In the following years, it was seen that the loss of the kidney function could be reduced from 10 to 5 ml/min per year, i.e. the loss could be halved.

The clinical importance of this was enormous. The known and short survival term of 7 years could be extended to 14 years. The evidence level was not high – a not very convincing 3.

Nevertheless, the treatment established itself – and quite rightly – all around the world. The final proof was produced only many years later in much larger studies, as described below. In the intervening years, many thousand patients had benefited from the aggressive blood pressure lowering treatment that was introduced after the early small studies

Blocking the renin-angiotensin system

In the following years, a number of new principles were developed for blood pressure lowering treatment. In the mid-1980s, it became possible to lower blood pressure with new drugs that could block the renin-angiotensin system. This led to a large number of studies carried out under the auspices of the same research groups. As a rule, the design of the studies was the same. All patients were given everything there was in the medicine cupboard to lower blood pressure, and then they were randomized to also being given a pill that blocked the renin-angiotensin system. The investigated groups were often small, rarely larger than 100. Nevertheless, results were again found indicating that there was an extra advantage in using these new principles for treatment. Once again, the treatments swept all before them even though the formal evidence level was low. This was so because the studies did not have statistical strength to show an effect at the most important clinical end-points: cardiovascular diseases, kidney failure and death. In recent years, major GCP studies have remedied this situation and shown that blocking the renin-angiotensin system either by ACE inhibitors or by angiotensin II antagonists has a special effect over and beyond the blood pressure lowering effect. In September 2001, three such studies (called IRMA, IDNT and RENAAL respectively) were published in the same issue of the New England Journal of Medicine with Hans-Henrik Parving as co-author of two of them. The same good effect was demonstrated in the LIFE study and the evidence level for the effect on morbidity and death has been raised to level 1.

We no longer believe. We know!

Today, it is discussed whether there is a difference if one blocks the renin-angiotensin system with an Angiotensin Converting Enzyme (ACE) inhibitor or the receptor (A II-antagonists). Many studies at a low evidence level indicate that there is a difference. The only study that has directly compared the groups of substances shows that there is not. Also this study has a Dane, Professor Sten Madsbad, as co-author.

Lipid-lowering treatment

Even though it was known for many years that especially patients with type 2 diabetes could have dyslipidaemia, including hypercholesterolaemia, it was until relatively recently entirely unclarified whether there was any meaning at all in treating cholesterol lipid metabolism. This was very much due to the fact that there were no effective drugs available. With the entry of the statins into the arena, it became possible to test whether cholesterol-lowering treatment could give results. I have already described the so-called Heart Protection Study. This was an investigator-initiated study, run by a group of independent researchers from Oxford, UK. The study was ambitious and comprised 20,000 patients. The design was interesting, since it randomized patients with cholesterol levels that were judged by the patients' usual physicians to be acceptable. In other words, the physicians had not found an indication for treatment. The study showed with convincing strength that the treatment was effective. Morbidity and mortality were markedly reduced in the treated group. The effect was largest in the group of patients who also had diabetes. The evidence level is 1.

We no longer believe. We know!

Multifactorial intervention

In 2003, a new Steno Study was published from Steno Diabetes Center. This was a clinically controlled randomized trial of the effect of multiple intervention conventional treatment. This is an excellent example of the possibilities an institution like Steno Diabetes Center has for conducting an important study, even with the heightened demands that are made today of clinically controlled trials. The Steno 2 Study investigated the effect on cardiovascular disease and mortality of a mixed package of diet, glycaemic regulation, blood pressure lowering treatment with an ACE inhibitor, statin treatment, other drug intervention, smoking cessation and various lifestyle changes. The treatment package worked on patients with type 2 diabetes, and the evidence level is high. Also this study, together with UKPDS and the Heart Protection Study, has led to changes in all guidelines for treatment of patients with type 2 diabetes.

We no longer believe. We know!

A little more about guidelines

The object of guidelines is to recommend treatments that can improve patients' clinical situation/health. In the field of diabetes, there are many guidelines today. Ideally, they would be based on the highest evidence levels, i.e. 2 and preferably 1. In practice, this is rarely the case. As I have described the situation, there are high evidence levels for the importance of glycaemic regulation, blood pressure lowering treatment, blocking of the renin-angiotensin system and for statin treatment. Many other factors are included in the guidelines.

There are often many studies in these fields, but they are usually at the lower evidence level of 3 or perhaps even 4. This might, for example, apply to the effect of physical activity (which is, however, now well documented), diet, social status, mental status, smoking, obesity, but it could also apply to the effect of, for instance, patient education, self-care, and whatever other concepts are attached to patient treatment. Can one use such guidelines, which are based on evidence levels 3 and 4? Of course one can. Precisely that type of evidence will often have been discussed at consensus conferences, at which the objective is to reach agreement on recommendations of treatments against the background of the available, often modest, evidence. The most important thing for the individual therapist is that one should judge the strengths and weaknesses of guidelines on the basis of an overall assessment of the evidence level. This will often lead to the critical questions that may in turn lead to further research and development.

Afterthought

There is still room for sensible clinical judgements. I will end with an example. Patients in a phase with progressive renal failure are treated today as I have described. Then there comes a time when the patient can no longer manage without dialysis treatment. The patient reaches a stage in his or her disease where one does not know if there is still any effect at all of the ongoing treatment. For dialysis patients, the effect of the described multifactorial intervention is virtually undocumented. Should the lack of documentation for dialysis patients mean that the treatment that functioned at a high evidence level prior to dialysis should be interrupted? In reality, we don't know. Many nephrologists think that the treatment is superfluous once the patient is in dialysis. For my own part, I have on this question made the choice to maintain the already established treatment until the day comes when it is proved that it is harmful.

I don't know. I believe!

Do I, nevertheless, believe in the value of EBM? – Yes, EBM has come to stay.

SUPPLEMENTARY READING:

Deckert T, Poulsen JE. Diabetic nephropathy: Fault or Destiny? Diabetologia 1981;21:178-83

Wulff HR. Rationel Klinik. Grundlaget for diagnostiske og terapeutiske beslutninger. 1. ed. Copenhagen: Munksgaard, 1973

Wulff HR, Gøtzsche PC. Rational Diagnosis and Treatment. Oxford: Blackwell 1976, 1981 and 2000

Parving HH, Andersen AR, Smidt UM, Svendsen PA. Early aggressive antihypertensive treatment reduces rate of decline in kidney function in diabetic nephropathy. Lancet 1983; i:1175-9

Brenner BM, Copper ME, de Zeeuw D, Keane WF, Mitch WE, Parving HH, Remuzzi G, Snapinn SM, Zhang Z, Shahinfar S. Effects of losartan on renal and cardiovascular outcomes in patients with type 2 diabetes and nephropathy. N Engl J with 2001;345:861-9

Parving HH, Lehnert H, Bröchner-Mortensen J, Gomis R, Andersen S, Arner P. Effect of irbesartan on the development of diabetic nephropathy in patients with type 2 diabetes, N Engl J with 2001;345:870-8

Feldt-Rasmussen B, Mathiesen ER, Deckert T. Effect of two years of strict metabolic control on progression of incipient nephropathy in insulin-dependent diabetes. Lancet 1986;ii:1300-4

Wang PH, Lau J, Chalmers TC. Meta-analysis of effects of intensive blood-glucose control on late complications of type 1 diabetes. Lancet 1993;341:1306-9

The Diabetes Control and Complications Trial Research Group. The effect of intensive treatment of diabetes on the development and progression of long-term complications in insulin-dependent diabetes mellitus. N Engl J with 1993;329:977-86

Gæde P, Vedel P, Larsen N, Jensen GVH, Parving HH, Pedersen O. Multifactorial intervention and cardiovascular disease in patients with type 2 diabetes. N Engl J with 2003;348:383-93

MRC/BHF heart protection study of cholesterol lowering with simvastatin in 20.536 high-risk individuals: a randomised placebo-controlled trial. Lancet 2002;360:7-22

Clinical Practice Recommendations 2005, American Diabetes Association. Diabetes Care 2005;28(suppl 1)

TYPE 1 DIABETES – THE COPENHAGEN MODEL

THOMAS MANDRUP-POULSEN

What is the Copenhagen Model?

The Copenhagen Model "classic" was first published in this form in 1987 [1], although a very early version can be said to have seen the light of day already in 1986 [2]. The model integrates our knowledge of the progression of the disease that leads to insulin-dependent diabetes, now designated type 1 diabetes.

The model assumes that this process takes place islet by islet, which helps to explain that the inflammatory process that leads to type 1 diabetes is desynchronized in time and space, i.e. it takes place over a long period and not in all islets at the same time, and that inflammation is seen only in islets where there are beta-cells.

The model implicates that the beta-cell destruction is not beta-cell specific. The other hormone-producing cells in the islet of Langerhans are exposed to the same signal substances, but only beta-cells are destroyed because of inherent properties attached to their specialized function that make them particularly sensitive to the effect of cytokines. In this way, the model moves the focus from the contemporary view of the role of the immune system as an indiscriminate killer to a perception of the beta-cell as playing an active role in its own destruction: the beta-cell dies because it is a beta-cell [3]. This response of a beta-cell is unique opening the possibility for developing drugs that affect the signalling pathways activated by cytokines in the beta-cell, but not in other cells. The T-cells do not, then, kill the beta-cells directly through contact-dependent killer mechanisms, but the most important role of the T-cells is to focus, orchestrate and amplify the inflammatory process in the islet of Langerhans.

Finally, the model seeks to explain that the occurrence of type 1 diabetes is not genetically restricted by certain tissue type genes (HLA genes), even though the disease is closely linked with certain genes in the HLA region. This absence of an HLA restriction is a precondition for the possibility

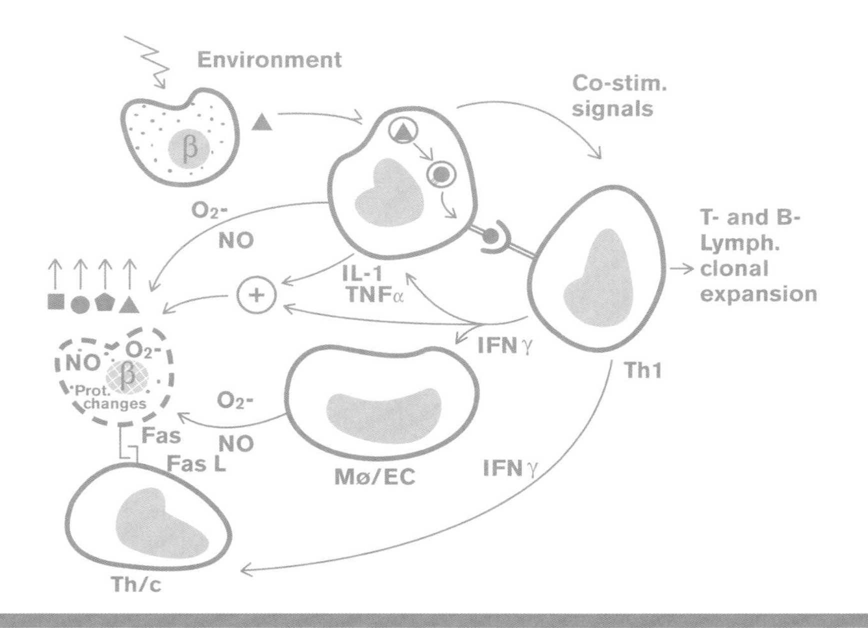

The Copenhagen Model of type 1 diabetes in 1994.

that all natural or changed beta-cell antigens and thereby a range of environmental factors could in principle be imagined to trigger the disease. The predisposing genes hereby seem to play more of a quantitative than a qualitative role in the reaction of the immune system to the beta-cells.

Criticism and acceptance

The model has encountered criticism, especially from immunologists who on the basis of studies of the spontaneously diabetic animal model, the NOD mouse, have claimed that beta-cell killing *is* specific, as T-cells are the central killer cells through cell-to-cell contact-dependent killer mechanisms. This view is not, however, in agreement with observations in, for example, the NOD mouse, to the effect that none of the T-cell-dependent killing mechanisms are indispensable in the disease process. Twenty years after the model was presented, widespread agreement has gradually developed that the inflammatory and the T-cell-specific disease models supplement each other, and that both mechanisms may very well be involved [4].

The discovery that cytokines are beta-cell toxic [5] is a central precondition in the Copenhagen Model, and the prehistory of and the course of events in this discovery will be briefly described below.

Background

Scientific discoveries rarely, if ever, come out of the blue. Ideas rest on a synthesis of already existing knowledge and the application of technological breakthroughs; a fruitful research environment; and the necessary resources, including a motivated team of researchers, often made up of members recruited from outside the core research area.

In June 1971, Jørn Nerup published an article in *Diabetes* [6], which was a logical continuation of his dissertation from 1969 on corresponding findings in patients with Addison's disease. This work is regarded by many as the starting point for the research effort that has made it possible to classify juvenile diabetes as an immune-mediated disease.

The article in *Diabetes* showed for the first time in diabetes patients cell-mediated immune reactivity *in vitro* and *in vivo* to homogenates of foetal calf pancreas or pancreatic tissue isolated from pigs. The porcine tissue was enriched in hormone-forming tissue by ligating the duct, so that the part of the gland that forms digestive enzymes is destroyed. The choice of this technique was inspired by a corresponding method used 50 years previously by Banting and Best and others before them in efforts to isolate the blood glucose regulating hormone. The interventions in Danish Landrace pigs were performed in a barn at Jacob E Poulsen's brother-in-law's farm in Tølløse, where Nerup anaesthetized the animals with a primitive ether mask, while Ole Ortved Andersen operated and Gunnar Bendixen kept curious spectators at a distance. The animals survived, and islet-enriched tissue could later be harvested. Subsequent operations, which were performed in the Ferrosan building in Blegdamsvej with professional help from Rigshospitalet's anaestheticians and gastroenterological surgeons, were unfortunate: all the animals died.

The leucocyte migration method

Nerup and his team had already realized at this time that the migration inhibition of leucocytes had to be mediated by soluble factors secreted from the activated lymphocytes, so-called lymphokines. The factor inhibiting migration was designated the *Migration Inhibitory Factor*, MIF. At this time, none of these factors had been characterized biochemically, but were designated on the basis of their activity in a relevant biological assay. This circumstance gave rise to considerable scepticism on the part of cellular immunologists, who collectively designated lymphokines as *lymphodreck*, until at the end of the 1970s and the beginning of the 1980s, these factors were purified, characterized, and cloned.

An early project proposal

In a project proposal dated November 1972, Nerup puts forward a hypothesis on behalf of a project group also including Claes Hellerström, Uppsala University, who was the first to isolate the islets of Langerhans by microdissection, and Gunnar Bendixen. It ran: *"Lymphocytes that infiltrate the islet tissue in juvenile diabetics can be imagined to release lymphokines. What effect do lymphokines have on beta-cells?"*

The protocol described how lymphocytes isolated from a patient with powerful cell-mediated immune reactivity to calf pancreas, demonstrated by the leucocyte migration test (LMT), were to be exposed to this antigen. The liquid phase (the supernatant) over the cells was to be isolated and sent by plane to Uppsala, where it was to be added to islet cultures with a view of investigating their effects on *"the measurable metabolic parameters in connection with the function of the beta-cells"* and *"... the islet ultrastructure assessed by electron microscopy"*.

In a letter dated 6.12.1972 to Rolf Gunnarsson, Histological Department, Uppsala University, Nerup writes in answer to comments on the protocol of 24.11.1972 among other things: *"We have now developed the necessary method for MIF production and expect to start the first trial on 12.12.72. Isolated lymphocytes + monocytes from a patient who has reacted well in the leucocyte migration test will be incubated with foetal calf pancreas and foetal calf liver and also put into control cultures without addition of antigen. We will freeze the supernatants in small ampoules and be ready to send them to you ... (with a view of) ...testing the supernatants in various dilutions on the islets with release of insulin and insulin synthesis investigations."*

Trials with cells from 3-4 more patients and controls were planned before Christmas 1972.

Why did these experiments not materialize?

Concurrently with these plans, Nerup and his colleagues were working on another series of experiments/studies performed on mice, which were primitively and discreetly housed in the archive under pavilion E4 at Frederiksberg Hospital. Based on the hypothesis that environmental factors such as viruses could contribute to triggering diabetes by activating cell-mediated immunity to virus-infected beta-cells, Nerup and his colleagues had shown that mice infected with EMC virus (encephalomyocarditis virus), a virus that provokes experimental inflammation of the brain and of the heart muscle in mice, developed impaired glucose tolerance. As appears from the letter cited above, there were however considerable difficulties in reproducing these preliminary findings. This was frustrating for the group because it had not been possible to obtain sufficient test animals to investigate whether the effect was due to an effect on the beta-cells. Nerup got the idea that the difference in response to EMC virus infection was due to genetic variation. These considerations led Nerup and his group to examine the association between the HLA system and juvenile diabetes and to publish in 1974.

So the answer to the question why the supernatant experiments that had been planned in detail were not carried out at this time as projected, must essentially be that other projects had to be given priority. Furthermore, Nerup was engaged at this time in completing the survey article for his doctoral thesis during a stay with Rolf Luft in Stockholm.

A troublesome start

These ideas were however not forgotten. On being appointed to a post as Registrar at Steno Memorial Hospital, I became involved in a number of studies in Nerup's group. From February 1984, I obtained a research fellowship from the Michaelsen Foundation with a view to studying cell-mediated antipancreatic immunity in patients with newly diagnosed type 1 diabetes and islet-cell antibody-positive first-degree relatives with the help of LMT and islet-antigen from calves. In continuation of the proud tradition of rural experiments, Jens Høiriis-Nielsen and I made an agreement with a North Zealand farmer that we could remove the pancreas from newly slaughtered calves. Because the conditions were primitive, and because I lacked any kind of abdominal surgical expertise, while Jens Høiriis fully lived up to the example set by Gunnar Bendixen in mainly restricting himself to giving good advice (*"Thomas, you must operate. You know I' m not a doctor!"*), we did not succeed in isolating sufficient antigen in this way. Furthermore, as we did not manage to freeze immune cells without unspecifically stimulating MIF activity, and as LMT failed to work as it should, at the end of April 1984, I was miserably obliged to recognize that the methodical preconditions for the first four sub-protocols could not be fulfilled and that the major part of my doctoral thesis project could not be implemented as planned.

The first experiments

I was now urged by Nerup and Klaus Bendtzen to test the last sub-protocol: the effect of lymphokines on the islets of Langerhans. Here the methodical preconditions were fulfilled: At Hagedorn Research Laboratory Høiriis-Nielsen had established the islet-isolation method and had in his doctoral dissertation analyzed in detail the culture conditions and functional studies

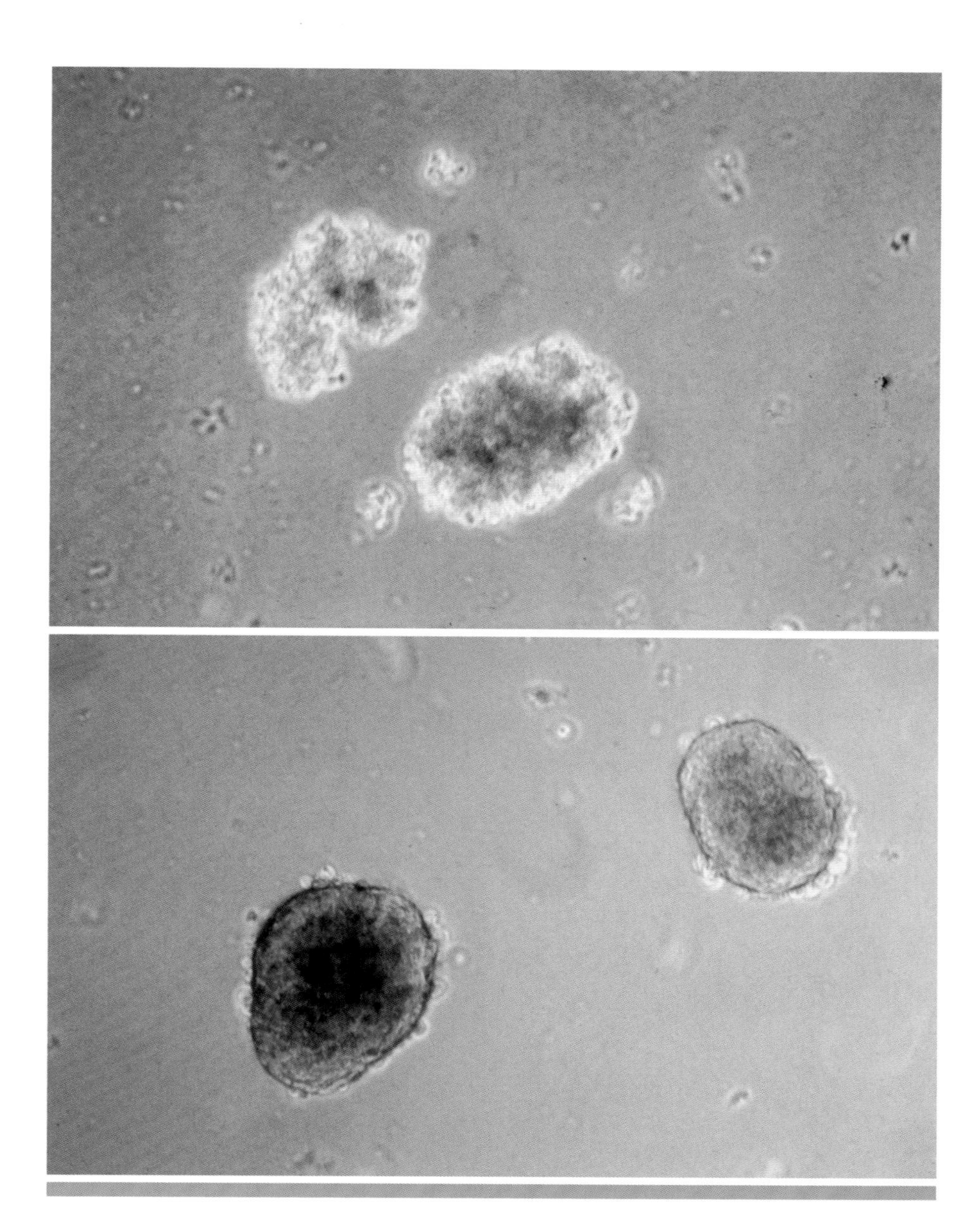

"The first attempt". Bottom: intact isolated rat islets in cultures with added supernatant from unstimulated white blood cells. Top: isolated rat islets with added supernatants from healthy normal persons' white blood cells stimulated with a mitogen (PHA). The islets are on their way to total disintegration. A shocking observation with very considerable consequences for the understanding of the pathogenesis in type 1 diabetes. (Data from the author).

with pertaining assays for hormone secretion and DNA content as surrogates for cell viability. Furthermore, Bendtzen had frozen and freeze-dried supernatants in stock, ready to be tested. These tests were quickly planned together with Høiriis-Nielsen. While on 8.5.1984 I was occupied with re-fishing calf islets from the isolation and on 9.-10.5 with measuring insulin and amylase on the tissue, I had agreed with Jens that his laboratory technicians Ragna Jørgensen and Dagny Jensen should set up the first experiments with islets from adult rats isolated by our group of students on 9.5. and harvest them on 16.5. In order to reproduce these tests, every Wednesday laboratory technician Susanne Grinderslev and I isolated rat islets that had to be pre-cultered for 7 days, set up in experiment and harvested after 7 days. When I was going to harvest islets for the first time in the dissection microscope after 7 days' exposure to supernatant, I noticed a strikingly changed morphology of the islets exposed to supernatant from stimulated cells: the islets were almost dissolved! I was enthusiastic and asked Åke Lernmark, head of research at Hagedorn Research Laboratory, who was passing by, to have a look. Åke tended to think that I should make sure that it was not PHA (phytohemagglutinin)/tuberculin that had been used to stimulate the cells, which was harmful to the islets. I set up control experiments that showed that it was not these stimuli that influenced the islets. In September 1984, we were so sure of the effects on rat islets that we decided to test supernatants on human islets. The experiment was set up on 7.9.1984 and confirmed the effects on the rat islets, although the human islets were a little less sensitive.

Our work was presented for the first time at the European Society for Clinical Investigation, Toulouse, on 24.-27.4.1985 [7]. We had difficulties in getting the work accepted for publication. A general criticism was that the effect was after all rather unspecific, since the supernatants were produced by stimulating the mononuclear cells of healthy persons with antigen-unspecific methods. So how could this be relevant? Our counter-arguments to the effect that what was revolutionarily new was precisely that the effector mechanism was unspecific, while the specificity was conditioned by T-lymphocyte-dependent focusing of the inflammation to the islets of Langerhans and by the beta-cells' unique sensitivity to these mediators made no impression at all, and we ended up publishing in *Allergy* [5]. Gunnar Bendixen consoled me by saying that it doesn't matter where one publishes as long as the work is good, and Jacob E Poulsen assured me that the verdict of history is just.

The identification of the active principle: interleukin-1

Our expectation based on the first studies was that we would have to look for a T-cell factor, and we therefore tested the effect of a number of accessible purified cytokines on islets, four of which were lymphokines (IL-2, lymphotoxin, LIF (leucocyte migration inhibitory factor) and MIF), while only one was a monokine: interleukin-1. At the time when we set up the first experiment on 20.02.1985, only IL-2 and IL-1 were cloned, and there were no recombinantly produced available cytokines. We found that only IL-1 was able to reproduce the effects of the supernatants, and to be sure of the IL-1-effects, we tested 2 batches of purified IL-1 and a preparation of proIL-1 procured by Charles A Dinarello, at that time at Tufts University School of Medicine in Boston, and later a close friend and collaborator. We had to conclude that the macrophage as the most important source of IL-1 could be an important effector cell. This was an emerging principle at the time. In 1984, Ed Leiter's group in the USA had shown that activated macrophages were toxic for islet cells, but the killing mechanism had not been demonstrated.

Our early findings were mentioned by Nerup in an invited lecture at the IDF meeting in Madrid in September 1985. Our data were criticised for not excluding the possibility that impurities in the purified preparations might be the cause of the results. It was therefore now crucial to show that recombinantly produced IL-1 could reproduce these findings, and that neutralization of IL-1 blocked the toxic effect of the supernatants. In experiments in which I was blinded in relation to the content of the preparations we received from Dinarello's laboratory, we were able to show just that, and that the quantities that influenced islet function were precisely the quantities that activated T-cells, i.e. pathophysiologically relevant concentrations. We prepared this study for submission to *Nature*.

Models, hypotheses – and tensions

Things now began to accelerate. We needed time to discuss trials, results, interpretations and models, and we needed a pathogenetic model that placed the macrophage and IL-1 in relation to other observations concerning effector functions and beta-cell destruction.

On 3-4.9.1985, a group consisting of Nerup, Høiriis-Nielsen, Jens Mølvig, Giatgen Spinas, Birgit Sehested Hansen and the present writer visited Nerup's converted farmhouse by Lake Bolmen in Småland, Sweden. Here we discussed how our observations fitted in with the prevailing pathogenetic view, and where they gave occasion for a change of paradigm. These observations and hypotheses were summed up in a note ("The Bolmen Note"), also in graphic form, that formed the basis for the Copenhagen

Model. The note gave rise to tensions between Nerup and Bendtzen, for in a handwritten letter from Nerup to Bendtzen dated 10.10.1985, Nerup writes, among other things: "*... Thanks also for the comments on "the Bolmen Note". We may disagree on the interpretation of certain hypotheses and observations, but otherwise I don't think we disagree particularly. Nor that "credit" should be shared everywhere. ... It's probably a good idea if we find time for a thorough discussion of these matters, and of the division of labour and roles as "first author". There can hardly be any major problems in this. The matter is more important than persons. ... The observations are too exciting and the collaboration too good to let "noise" disturb us ...*".

At the time when the draft article for *Nature* was to be formulated, I was engaged in writing two papers: one on the identification of IL-1 based on screening of purified activities, later published in *Diabetologia* 1986, and one that described a number of necessary control and characterization trials, later published in *Allergy* 1986. The agreement was therefore that Bendtzen would write the draft for *Nature*. The article was rejected there, but was then sent to *Science*, which accepted the work [8]. Unfortunately, Nerup and Bendtzen broke off their collaboration in 1987.

The first review paper that presented a model view of these findings was published in 1986 [2]. The model contained a number of the elements of the Copenhagen Model, but was not yet fully developed.

Further phenomenological and mechanistic studies

A critical issue related to the role of IL-1 in the pathogenesis of Type 1 diabetes was the beta-cell specificity. In the previous studies, we had observed effects on both insulin and glucagon secretion. It was therefore important to clarify whether the *cytotoxic* effect was beta-cell specific. In collaboration with Jørn Egeberg at Institute of Medical Anatomy B, University of Copenhagen, we carried out blinded quantitative morphological studies of the ultrastructure of rat islets and human islets using electron microscopy after exposure to IL-1. Laboratory technician Trine Grainger performed the laborious embeddings and sectioning. We could show that the toxic effect was beta-cell specific, that human islets required longer exposure, and that the morphological findings indicated that the beta-cells perished through apoptosis, a sort of programmed cell death. The work was sent to *Diabetologia*, which however rejected it with the argument that it contained "split-data" from the *Science* article, which was incorrect: all the experiments were performed after submission of the *Science* study. It was subsequently published in *APMIS*.

Even though immunoadsorption of supernatants neutralized their beta-cell toxic effect, we could not disregard the possibility that other in themselves inactive cytokines might potentiate the effect of IL-1. We therefore tested IL-1 in combination with a number of other cytokines and were able to show that for example TNF and IL-6 potentiated the effects of IL-1, and others showed that this was also the case for IFN, a finding we missed because we used human IFN on rat islets.

Now followed a long series of further studies to explain the effects of the cytokines on the beta-cell in our and other laboratories. Heated academic discussions arose, many probably based on differences in experimental conditions: was IL-1 toxic only for purified beta-cells? Could IL-1 alone kill human beta-cells? There is however agreement today that the combination of IL-1 and IFN/TNF triggers beta-cell death in isolated islets from all investigated species. The signalling *cross-talk* between these cytokines has been only partially mapped, just as the charting of the genes that are decisive for the development of the beta-cell's special sensitivity to cytokines has only just begun. We still lack genetic animal models in which the receptors for IL-1 and IFN/TNF have been knocked out in order to test the model fully *in vivo*. Furthermore, there is a need for more studies of human tissue sections from islets infiltrated with monocytic cells with a view to the cytokines' role.

Conclusion

The papers briefly described here, published between the middle of 1985 and the end of 1987, formed the nucleus of the classical Copenhagen Model. In the following 20 years, we and many other groups have worked to describe the phenomenology and mechanisms of the beta-cell cytotoxic effect, to understand the signalling pathways and intracellular effector mechanisms that induce beta-cell apoptosis and to test the hypothesis in animal models. Together with proteome- and transcriptome-analyses, the model has served as a source of candidate genes for genetic association and linkage studies and for the first attempts at mathematically describing a pathophysiological system as a dynamic instability.

There are still many questions that the Copenhagen Model has not answered: what triggers antigen release from the beta-cells? What proteins become antigenic and why? What factors attract the macrophages to the islets? What circumstances break peripheral T-cell tolerance and regulation? Why is the human islet less sensitive than rat islets? What makes the beta-cell especially sensitive to cytokine toxicity in relation to other cells? Why is the pathogenetic process retarded in certain individuals leaving a residual beta-cell function even after many years of diabetes? What is the role of cytokines in humans in the development of type 1 diabetes?

There is a great need for clinical studies of diabetes patients with substances that inhibit IL-1 and the biological effects of other cytokines. The time is now ripe for this, since anti-IL-1-treatment on the basis of experience from the treatment of more than 100,000 patients with rheumatoid arthritis seems to be very safe, and a number of anti-IL-1-principles are being developed with high affinity to IL-1 or the IL-1 receptor, which can be administered with intervals stretching from weeks to months. *Proof-of-principle* that anti-IL-1 treatment can protect the beta-cell function in humans derives from a recent clinical study we carried out with Marc Donath in Zürich in type 2 diabetes [9], where on the basis of studies from human islets *in vitro*, the mechanism seems to be that glucose induces IL-1-production from the beta-cells, and that an autocrine effect of IL-1 on the beta-cells triggers signals for cell death that are very reminiscent of those that are activated when IL-1 is produced as part of an inflammatory process because of immune-cell infiltration in the islets in type 1 diabetes. In other words, both metabolic and inflammatory stimuli seem able to trigger beta-cell death by converging on the same molecular mechanisms.

There are further clinical studies in the pipeline for both type 1 and 2 diabetes, and in the coming years, it will become clear whether the Copenhagen Model can maintain its relevance, should be substantially revised or has to be rejected entirely. There is a need for new models and hypotheses that can challenge the Copenhagen Model, which after 20 years in its by and large unchanged form risks becoming just as dogmatic and uncritically accepted as the models that it once attacked.

REFERENCES

1. *Nerup J, Mandrup-Poulsen T, Mølvig J, Spinas G, Nielsen JH, Dinarello CA, Hansen BS, Palme JP. Pathogenesis of insulin-dependent diabetes mellius (IDDM). In: Christiansen C, Riis BJ, eds. Highlights on Endocrinology. Proceedings of the First European Congress on Endocrinology, Copenhagen, June 21-25, 1987. Viborg: Nørhaven 1987:37-41*
2. *Nielsen JH, Mandrup-Poulsen T, Spinas GA, Hansen BS, Mølvig J, Nerup J, Bendtzen K (1986) Possible role of interleukin 1 (IL-1) in the pathogenesis of insulin-dependent diabetes mellitus (IDDM) In: Jaworsky, MA, Molnar GD,*

Rajotte RV, Singh B, eds. The immunology of diabetes mellitus. Amsterdam, New York, Oxford: Exerpta Medica 1986:95-103

3. *Nerup J, Mandrup-Poulsen T, Helquist S, Andersen HU, Pociot F, Reimers JI, Cuartero BG, Karlsen AE, Bjerre U, Lorenzen T. On the pathogenesis of IDDM. Diabetologia 1994;37[suppl.1]:82-9*
4. *Mathis D, Vence L, Benoist C. ß-cell death during progression to diabetes. Nature 2001;414:792-8*
5. *Mandrup-Poulsen T, Bendtzen K, Nielsen JH, Bendixen G, Nerup J. Cytokines cause functional and structural damage to isolated islets of Langerhans. Allergy 1985;40:424-9*
6. *Nerup J, Andersen OA, Bendixen G, Egeberg J, Poulsen JE. Antipancreatic cellular hypersensitivity in diabetes mellitus. Diabetes 1971;20:424-7*
7. *Mandrup-Poulsen T, Grinderslev S, Bendtzen K, Nielsen JH, Bendixen G, Nerup J. Soluble blood mononuclear cell mediators cause functional and structural damage to isolated islets of Langerhans. 19th Annual Meeting of the European Society for Clinical Investigation, Toulouse, France, April 24-27, 1985. Abstract. Eur J Clin Invest 1985:15(part II):A2/9*
8. *Bendtzen K, Mandrup-Poulsen T, Nerup J, Nielsen JH, Dinarello CA, Svenson M. Cytotoxicity of human pI 7 interleukin-1 for pancreatic islets of Langerhans. Science 1986:232:1545-7*
9. *Larsen CM, Faulenbach M, Vaag A, Vølund A, Ehses JE, Seifert B, Mandrup-Poulsen T, Donath MY. Interleukin-1 receptor antagonist in type 2 diabetes mellitus. N Engl J Med 2007:356:1517-26*

GASTROINTESTINAL HORMONES – FROM CONCEPT TO TREATMENT

JENS JUUL HOLST

Historical background

The gastrointestinal hormone, secretin, was the first hormone to be discovered. This was in 1902 when the English physiologists Bayliss and Starling were able to produce pancreatic secretion in an anaesthetized dog by instillation – dripping in – of hydrochloric acid in a segment of the small intestine even though all the nerves from the segment were cut (the Russian physiologist Pavlov's experiments had led everyone to believe that sort of thing occurred via the nerves). They concluded that this therefore had to be *"a chemical reflex"*. An extract of the mucous membrane of the denerved segment also stimulated the pancreatic secretion: the first hormonal regulation was discovered, and the first "hormone" produced [1]. It was also Bayliss and Starling, who proposed the word hormone [2] from the Greek *"ὁρμάω"*, which means *"wakes to activity"*.

Later numerous other hormones appeared, not least from the gastrointestinal tract, which is the organ that produces the most hormones and has the most endocrine cells. A possible role for intestinal hormones in connection with diabetes was proposed already in 1906 by Moore [3], who tried to treat diabetes with extracts of duodenal mucous membrane. This did not work for him, but today, 100 years after Moore's attempt, treatment of type 2 diabetes based on a gastrointestinal hormone is a reality with a considerable clinical potential.

As early as around 1930, it became clear that there had to be a secretion from the intestine of hormones that affected the pancreas's regulation of the glucose metabolism, the so-called incretin hormones [4], and in 1964, it was directly shown that the insulin secretion – which could be measured after Berson and Yalow had developed the radioimmunoassay in 1959 – was stimulated more (up to four times as much) by oral glucose than by intravenous glucose. This was a sign of gastrointestinal hormones having stimulated the insulin secretion [5]. What hormones these might be was not known. The interest in intestinal and incretin hormones also spread to Denmark, and in 1972, Jens F Rehfeld, Claus Kühl and the present writer established a laboratory at Bispebjerg Hospital, devoted to research into these matters [6].

Intestinal glucagons

One of the original contributions from our group, which in time also came to include Jan Fahrenkrug and Ove Schaffalitzky de Muckadell, was the exclusion of the hormone secretin as a physiological incretin hormone [7]. The present writer's interest was focused on two peptides from the intestine that reacted with antibodies directed at the pancreas hormone, glucagon,

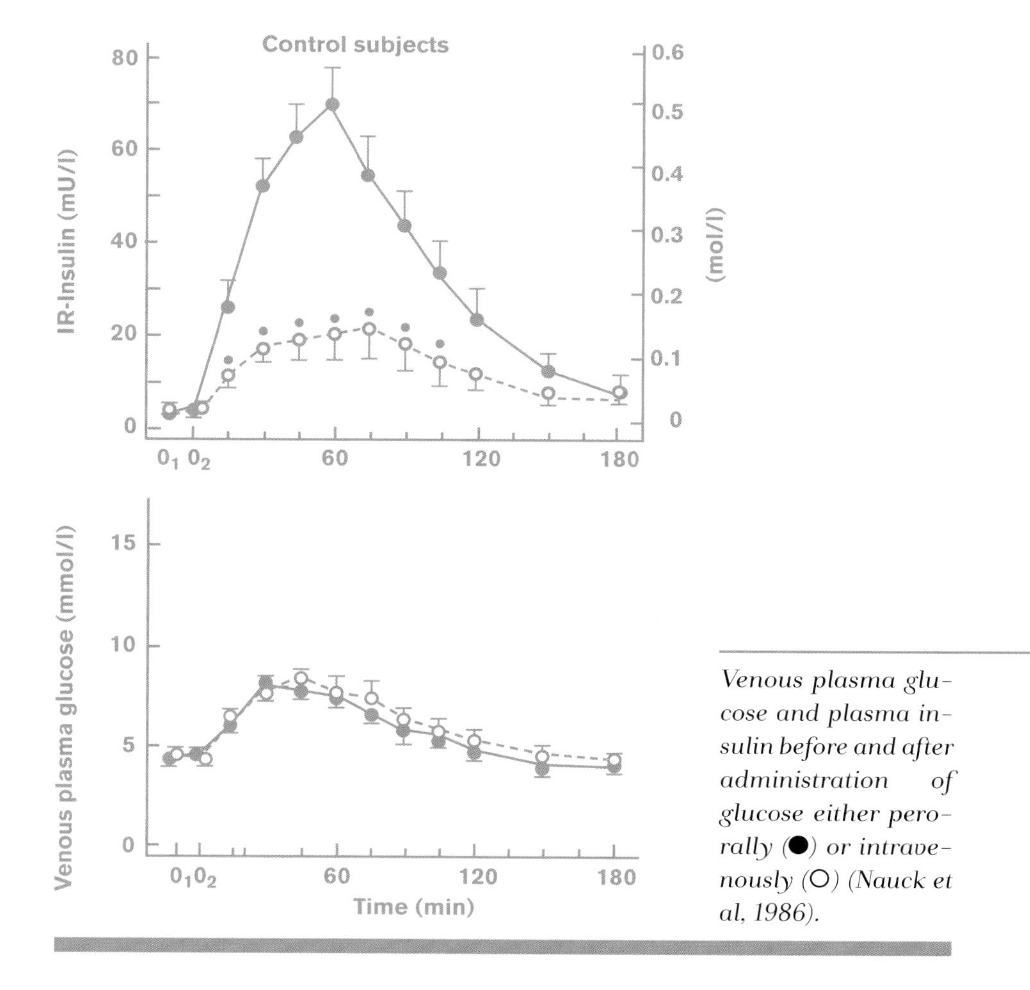

Venous plasma glucose and plasma insulin before and after administration of glucose either perorally (●) or intravenously (○) (Nauck et al, 1986).

but which were nevertheless clearly different from glucagon itself, the so-called intestinal glucagons. Using chromatographic and immunochemical methods, it proved possible to show that both peptides contained the entire glucagon sequence, which meant that they could be products of a larger precursor (proglucagon), that might perhaps be common to these "intestinal glucagons" and glucagon from the pancreas.

It was Lars Thim and Alistair Moody from Novo who elucidated the structure of the larger of the two intestinal glucagons [8]. They called it glicentin; it consists of 69 amino acids and contains, as expected, the entire 33 amino-acid glucagon molecule in positions 33-61. A little later, we were able to show that the other molecule, which is today called oxyntomodulin, was a fragment of glicentin corresponding to glucagon + the glicentin's 8 C-terminal amino acids. Oxyntomodulin, in fact, proved able to stimulate insulin secretion. Moreover, we found that a molecule corresponding to the first 30 amino acids of glicentin was secreted in parallel with glucagon from the pancreas, and thereby provided strong support for the theory

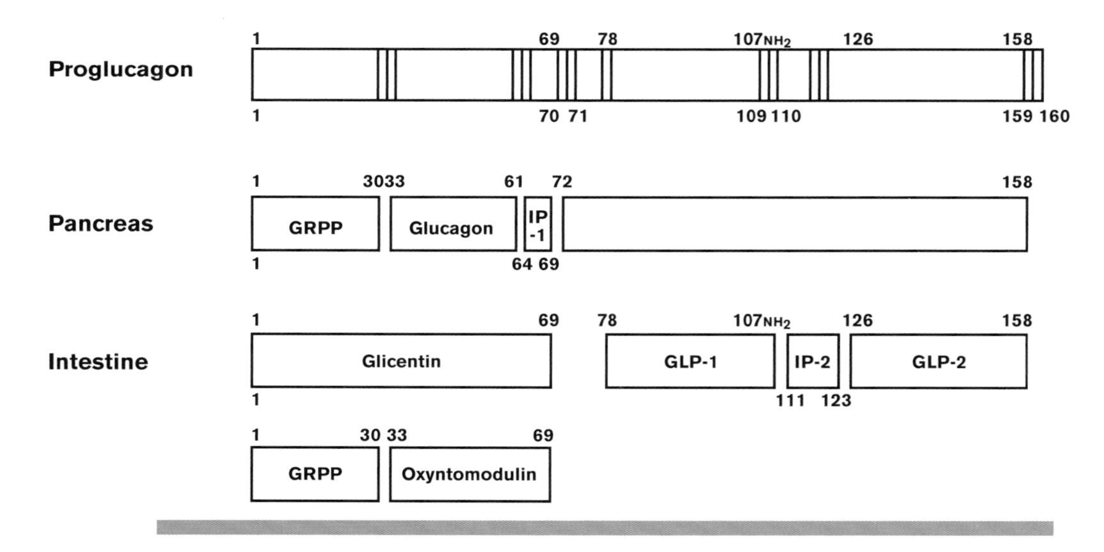

The structure of proglucagon and its split into glucagon, GLP-1 and GLP-2 in the pancreas and the intestinal membrane respectively. The figures give the placing of the amino acids in the 160-amino-acid-large prohormones. The vertical lines denote the placing of the basic amino acids (typical cleaving sites).
GRPP: Glicentin Related Pancreatic Polypeptide
IP: Intervening Peptide
NH_2 denotes that the C-terminal of GLP-1 is amidated.

of a common precursor [9]. However, various observations showed that proglucagon had to be much bigger than glicentin and contains a "*major proglucagon fragment*" without the glucagon sequence. It was Graeme Bell [10], who in 1983 using the new molecular-biological methods deduced the structure of the mRNA, which codes for the expression of proglucagon in hamster islets (and the structure of the human gene followed shortly after).

It is quite true that proglucagon first contains the glicentin sequence (in which glucagon is concealed), but in addition it also contains the precursor to two glucagon-like sequences (GLP-1 and GLP-2), which are flanked by a pair of basic amino acids. Such pairs are typically cleaving sites for pro-hormones. We immediately set about having the two glucagon-like peptides synthesized and developing measurement methods (radioimmunoassays) for both.

At the same time, we tested the peptides on our isolated, perfused porcine pancreas, but great was our disappointment when we saw that none of the substances affected the endocrine secretion. This was also surprising, because on the basis of examinations of patients with resections of various parts of the small intestine, we knew that a hormone had to be secreted with a powerful effect on the insulin secretion from the distal (lowest part of) small bowel, where most of the cells that produce glicentin are situated (the so-called L-cells). It could of course be oxyntomodulin, but analyses showed that the concentration of oxyntomodulin in the blood after oral glucose was probably too low to explain the incretin effect.

With our new analyses for GLP-1 and GLP-2, we therefore set about looking for the naturally occurring hormones in extracts of human and porcine intestines. We succeeded in isolating the natural GLP-1, which proved to be 6 amino acids shorter than predicted, and – what was no less important – it stimulated the insulin secretion from our isolated pancreas with unprecedented strength! A new incretin hormone had been found. At the same time, it was established that proglucagon splits differently depending on where it is expressed: in the pancreas, glucagon (+ the two flanking fragments) is formed, and in the intestine, on the other hand, glicentin, GLP-1 and GLP-2 (Cathrine Ørskov's dissertation project) [11]).

Parallel with these studies, we were also working on another peptide hormone from the intestine, namely GIP. GIP stands for gastric inhibitory polypeptide, and the peptide was isolated in 1973 by John Brown in Stockholm on the basis of these properties [12]. However, the substance proved to have a strong stimulating effect on the insulin secretion in various models and was therefore a strong incretin hormone candidate. The secretion and effect of GIP were the topics for dissertation projects for Keld Bernt Lauritsen [13] and Thure Krarup [14].

The studies pointed clearly to an important incretin effect of GIP in healthy persons but also showed that, as already mentioned, there had to be yet another incretin hormone that was secreted from the distal small intestine (GIP comes particularly from the proximal (upper part of the) small intestine). Unfortunately, it turned out that like glucose GIP had virtually no effect on the insulin secretion in patients with type 2 diabetes. This was extremely disappointing, and our enthusiasm when we stood with the new insulinotropic (insulin stimulating) hormone, GLP-1, in our hands, was indeed limited: it probably wouldn't work on the patients either.

However, in continued trials, we mapped the secretion and effect of GLP-1 in humans and experimental animals and made interesting finds. In contrast to GIP, GLP-1 proved to exercise a strong inhibitory effect on the glucagon secretion from the pancreas. This was interesting because – translated to *in vivo* circumstances – it might result in an inhibition of the liver's glucose production, which is of course inhibited by insulin and enhanced by glucagon. GLP-1 could therefore be imagined to reduce the blood glucose when fasting. Furthermore, we found that the GLP-1 effect on the insulin secretion was dependent on the glucose concentration and disappeared at concentrations just below normal fasting glucose concentration. Studies of humans confirmed the conflicting effects of the insulin and glucagon secretion and the inhibitory effect on the liver's glucose production, and showed also that despite these effects, one cannot evoke hypoglycaemia with GLP-1 because of the glucose-dependence of the effects.

Moreover, we found, again in humans, that GLP-1 had a strong inhibitory effect on motility and secretion in the gastrointestinal tract, not least on the evacuation speed of the stomach. A corresponding inhibition could be obtained by instillation in the distal small intestine of physiological quantities of lipid or carbohydrate, and parallel with this, a strong rise in the plasma concentration of GLP-1 was observed. GLP-1 therefore had to be regarded as participating in the physiological mechanism, which is called the "ileal brake", the endocrine inhibition of motility and secretion in the gastrointestinal tract, which is triggered by nutrients in the ileum (the small intestine), which perhaps signals that the absorptive capacity is now about to be reached. That the endogenous GLP-1 has these functions is today confirmed by trials with GLP-1 receptor antagonists in humans. In relation to diabetes, the finding was particularly interesting because administration of GLP-1 had to be expected to be able to reduce meal-related blood sugar increases via the effect on evacuation of the stomach.

Thus, GLP-1 functions as more than a classical incretin hormone, and it became relevant also to examine whether GLP-1 has effects on appetite and food intake, which are regulated by, among other things, hormones from precisely the gastrointestinal tract. GLP-1 proved to inhibit both.

Parallel with this, other groups showed that GLP-1 can affect the beta-cell mass in experimental animals [15]. Thus, GLP-1 evokes growth of beta-cells both in cultures and *in vitro*, and moreover promotes the new formation of beta-cells from precursor cells in the pancreatic ducts. And finally GLP-1 inhibits beta-cell apoptosis (programmed cell death), spontaneous and induced, in both human and murine (from mice) beta-cells.

Effect of GLP-1 in type 2 diabetes

There was thus every possible reason for investigating whether GLP-1 has a potential in the treatment of type 2 diabetes. In the first treatment trials, GLP-1 was infused in slightly supraphysiological doses for patients with type 2 diabetes, who were regulated by a *Biostator®*, an "artificial pancreas", which with the help of variable insulin and glucose infusions could keep the blood glucose more or less in place also in connection with meal intake. It turned out that the GLP-1 infusion could almost completely replace the amount of insulin that the *Biostator®* released in the control trials [16].

If this somewhat complicated protocol was perhaps not the best suited to illustrate GLP-1's potential in diabetes treatment, the subsequent demonstration that intravenous infusion of GLP-1 could completely normalize the fasting blood glucose in patients with severe long-duration type 2 diabetes was all the more convincing [17]. A further study gave the explanation of the discrepancy between the earlier GIP studies and the GLP-1 trials: using a hyperglycaemic clamp (blood glucose maintained at 9 mmol/l with intravenous infusion for both controls and patients) GLP-1 was able by and large to normalize the insulin secretion, while GIP was without effect. A normal inhibition of the glucagon secretion with GLP-1 was also obtained, while GIP was again without effect.

There was therefore every possible reason to seek to develop GLP-1 for diabetes treatment. One could expect: 1) stimulation of the insulin secretion without risk of hypoglycaemia; 2) inhibition of the glucagon secretion and thereby inhibition of the increased hepatic glucose production, which contributes to the increased fasting blood glucose in patients; 3) a reduction of the postprandial blood glucose fluctuations because of the effect of the stomach evacuation; 4) a loss of weight because of the effect on the appetite and food intake. Intravenous administration of GLP-1 was of course not a realistic treatment option in the longer term, but one could try subcutaneous injections.

All went well with injecting GLP-1 subcutaneously, the plasma concentration rose proportionally with the dose, but at doses above 1.5 nmol/ kg, nausea occurred and at yet higher doses vomiting. There was, then, a limit to how high one could go. Unfortunately, the highest tolerated dose had a very limited effect on the blood glucose, and the effect on the insulin secretion was short-lived. We measured the plasma concentrations of GLP-1 after the subcutaneous injection and found that the half-life was very short, about four minutes. But not just that, we also found from chromatographic analyses of plasma with GLP-1 added that the peptide was very rapidly degraded so that the 2 N-terminal amino acids are cut off, whereby the peptide is inactivated. The degradation could be inhibited completely by specific inhibitors of an enzyme dipeptidylpeptidase-4 (DPP-4), which therefore had to be responsible for the degradation. We therefore assumed that it was this enzyme that was to blame for the inactivation of GLP-1, also *in vivo*, and thereby for the short duration of the effect (Carolyn Deacon's dissertation project).

Clinical usefulness of GLP-1

It was therefore uncertain whether it was at all possible to treat type 2 diabetes with GLP-1. To investigate this in more detail, we decided after some introductory trials to carry out a 6-week treatment of type 2 patients with GLP-1 given as continuous subcutaneous infusion with the help of insulin pumps. The trial was carried out by Mette Zander at Hvidovre Hospital as part of her PhD thesis. Of 20 persons with rather severe type 2 diabetes and obesity, half were given GLP-1 and half salt water for 6 weeks. In the GLP-1 group, the blood glucose fell between 4 and 6 mmol/l, in both fasting blood glucose and 8-hour profiles; HbA_{1c} (glycated haemoglobin, a measurement of the average blood glucose concentration over a long period) fell by 1.3 %; the concentrations of free fatty acids in plasma fell; there was a significant weight loss of approx. 2 kg, probably in consequence of slightly reduced appetite, which was also measured; the beta-cell function, which was measured using a 30 mmol/l hyperglycaemic clamp and arginine infusion, was markedly improved; insulin sensitivity, which was measured using an euglycaemic, hyperinsulinaemic clamp, was almost doubled (assessed on the basis of the glucose infusion speed); and there were no adverse effects.

We had thus obtained a *"proof-of-concept"* for diabetes treatment based on the effects of GLP-1. One could now imagine that analogues of GLP-1 that were resistant to DPP-4 would be effective, and subsequent studies of analogues, in which amino acid no. 2 was replaced with other amino acids with small side chains, showed that the analogues were both effective in respect of insulin secretion and also survived much longer in test animals (pigs). The development of resistant analogues therefore had to be a viable path. There was, however, another possibility: namely inhibition of DPP-4 in analogy with the use of ACE-inhibitors in the hypertension treatment. Trials with pigs in our laboratory (now at the Panum Institute) with such inhibitors, which had already been developed in another context, showed that the inhibitors could completely prevent the degradation of infused GLP-1, which therefore caused a far larger insulin secretion.

Both the two possibilities for treatment, use of resistant GLP-1 analogues (so-called *incretin mimetics*) along with inhibitors of the enzyme DPP-4 (which are now called *incretin enhancers*) have now been developed to an extent that the first preparations are now on the market in certain countries, including the USA, and both were launched in Europe in the spring of 2007. Some of the trials that have formed the basis for the registration of the preparations have been published, and both treatment principles must be described as promising.

Incretin mimetics

The first registered preparation in this group is called *Byetta®* and is produced by Amylin Corporation in San Diego in collaboration with Lilly. This is a synthetic peptide (in its synthetic form called exenatide), which is identical to exendin-4, which was originally found in the saliva of a lizard from Arizona, the so-called Gila Monster (Heloderma Suspectum). As opposed to GLP-1, it is stable with DPP-4 and is also eliminated more slowly in the kidneys, which means that one can obtain relevant plasma concentrations for approx. 5 hours after subcutaneous injection of the maximum tolerable dose – exendin in large doses also causes nausea and vomiting. Treatment trials were therefore carried out, in which exenatide (synthetic exendin-4) was administered in this dose (10 µg) subcutaneously twice daily. In the clinical phase-3 trials, the substance was administered in addition to already existing but insufficient oral treatment.

In the course of 6 months, a clear fall was achieved in HbA_{1c}, from 8 to approx. 7 %, a recognized treatment goal, along with a significant loss of weight. In subsequent non-controlled open studies some of the patients have been followed for up to 3 years, and it appears that HbA_{1c} remains around the 7 %, while the weight loss continues at a slightly reduced rate, but not yet with a full levelling out of the weight curve. It is clear that *Byetta®*'s special advantage is the loss of weight. Unfortunately, it is not yet possible to say to what extent the effect also comprises a protection/proliferation of the beta-cells. If there had been a proliferative effect, one would have expected a falling rather than a constant concentration of HbA_{1c} as a sign of increased insulin secretion and therewith falling blood glucose. On the other hand, treatment with *Byetta®* twice daily covers only about 10 of the 24 hours, and it is possible that longer-lasting preparations will have a better effect. The constant HbA_{1c} could also be interpreted as beta-

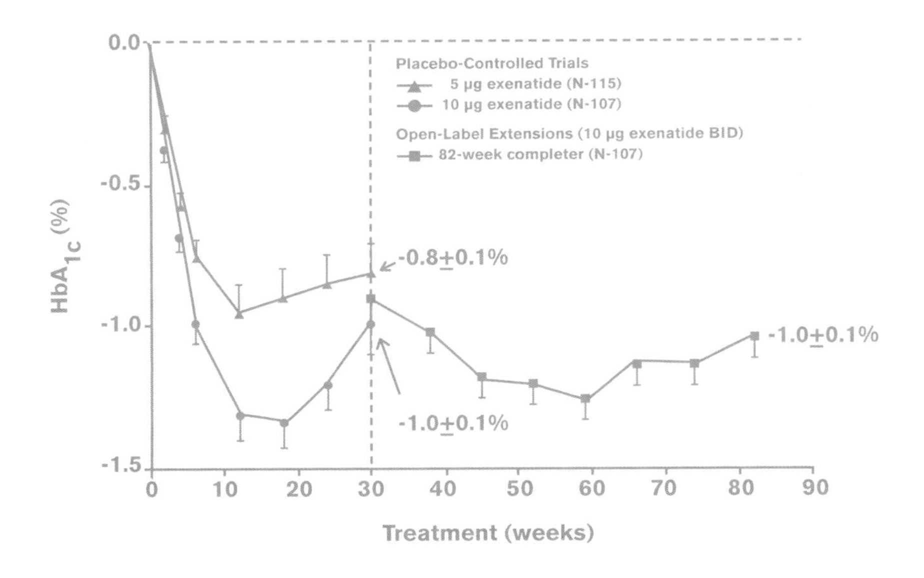

Change in HbA_{1c} during treatment with exenatide (Byetta®) *in relation to HbA_{1c} in placebo-treated patients with type 2 diabetes. (From Amylin's homepage).*

cell protection, since type 2 diabetes is of course progressive with falling beta-cell function and rising HbA_{1c}, which could well become evident over a period of 3 years. Unfortunately, there is no placebo group in the long-term studies mentioned. *Byetta*® gives rise to the formation of antibodies in a number of patients.

In Denmark, Novo Nordisk has developed a GLP-1 analogue, liraglutide, which is based on the structure of human GLP-1, to which a fatty acid is bound. Hereby liraglutide binds to albumin and achieves enzymatic stability and a long half-life (12 hours). Liraglutide can therefore be administered as single daily injections, which results in a relatively constant plasma level after 4-5 days. For this reason, liraglutide has few adverse effects, and it is only weakly antigenic. The clinical results (phase 2) with liraglutide comprise up to 2 % lowering of HbA_{1c}, a strong effect on fasting blood glucose and weight loss. Unfortunately, only results from treatments of 15 weeks' duration are accessible, but the phase-3 studies are approaching their conclusion.

Incretin enhancers (DPP-4 inhibitors)

Clinical trials with sitagliptin (trade name *Januvia*®) from MSD and with vildagliptin (Galvus, not yet approved) from Novartis, which are both publically accessible, have shown that with the chosen dose administered once daily almost 100 % inhibition of DPP-4 is achieved for most of the 24 hours. As a result of this, the concentration of intact GLP-1 (and GIP!) is increased by a factor of 2-3. The insulin secretion (e.g. at a test meal) is unchanged but at the same time the blood glucose falls so that the beta-cell's glucose sensitivity is improved. The glucagon secretion falls, where the opposite was expected because of the falling glucose concentration.

Phase-3 studies for both Galvus and *Januvia*® have shown an effect on HbA_{1c} corresponding to that obtained with *Byetta*®, both in monotherapy and in combination with other oral antidiabetic treatment. The effect has been seen to remain constant, at least for two years. As opposed to *Byetta*® and liraglutide, the inhibitors have no reducing effect on body weight, but they do not increase it either, which is clinically significant. Nor do they cause nausea, which is probably due to the fact that there are limits to how high concentrations of intact GLP-1 can be achieved with the inhibitors. No adverse effects have been identified that can be ascribed to the inhibition of DPP-4 or unspecific effects of the two inhibitors.

Conclusion

It can be concluded that both *incretin enhancers* and *incretin mimetics* represent new antidiabetic principles of treatment whose effect is at least comparable with that of existing preparations and which in combination with these result in improved metabolic regulation. The effect on body weight of *incretin mimetics* cannot be overestimated in consideration of the almost constant obesity that characterizes patients with type 2 diabetes. The low frequency of adverse effects using the inhibitors and the simple mode of administration tempt one to use these substances very early in the treatment of diabetes, perhaps even preventively in high-risk groups.

We have yet to see the real revolution in the treatment of diabetes, namely a protective effect on the beta-cells, but the results to date indicate that both groups have this potential.

So Moore was on the right track after all.

REFERENCES

1. *Bayliss W, Starling EH. Mechanism of pancreatic secretion. J Physiol (Lond) 1902;28:325-53*
2. *Starling EH. The chemical correlation of the functions of the body. The chemical control of the body. Croonian lecture. Lancet 1905;ii:338-41*
3. *Moore B, Edie ES, Abram JH. On the treatment of diabetes mellitus by acid extract of duodenal mucous membrane. Biochem J 1906;1:28-36*
4. *Zunz E, LaBarre J. Contributions a l'étude des variation physiologiques de la secretion interne de pancreas: relations entre les secretions externes et internes du pancreas. Archs Int Physiol Biochim 1929;31:20-44*
5. *McIntyre N, Holdsworth CD, Turner DS. New interpretation of oral glucose tolerance. Lancet 1964;ii:20-1*
6. *Rehfeld JF. Gastrointestinal hormones and insulin secretion. Scand J Gastroenterol 1972;7:289-92*
7. *Fahrenkrug J, Schaffalitzky de Muckadell OB, Kühl C. Effect of secretin on basal- and glucose-stimulated insulin secretion in man. Diabetologia 1978;14:229-34*
8. *Thim L, Moody AJ. The primary structure of porcine glicentin (proglucagon). Regul Pept 1981;2:139-50*
9. *Moody AJ, Holst JJ, Thim L, Jensen SL. Relationship of glicentin to proglucagon and glucagon in the porcine pancreas. Nature 1981;289:514-6*
10. *Bell GI, Santerre RF, Mullenbach GT. Hamster preproglucagon contains the sequence of glucagon and two related peptides. Nature 1983;302:716-8*
11. *Orskov C. Glucagon-like peptide-1, a new hormone of the entero-insular axis. Diabetologia 1992;35:701-11*
12. *Brown JC. Gastric inhibitory polypeptide. Monogr Endocrinol 1982;24:1-88*
13. *Lauritsen KB. GIP, incretin and gastrointestinal disease. Dan Med Bull 1983;30:204*
14. *Krarup T. Immunoreactive gastric inhibitory polypeptide. Endocr Rev 1988;9:122-34*
15. *Drucker DJ. Glucagon-like peptides: regulators of cell proliferation, differentiation, and apoptosis. Mol Endocrinol 2003;17:161-71*
16. *Gutniak M, Orskov C, Holst JJ, Ahren B, Efendic S. Antidiabetogenic effect of glucagon-like peptide-1 (7-36)amide in normal subjects and patients with diabetes mellitus [see comments]. N Engl J Med 1992;326:1316-22*
17. *Nauck MA, Kleine N, Orskov C, Holst JJ, Willms B, Creutzfeldt W. Normalization of fasting hyperglycaemia by exogenous glucagon-like peptide 1 (7-36 amide) in type 2 (non-insulin-dependent) diabetic patients. Diabetologia 1993;36:741-4*

FROM STEM CELL TO BETA-CELL – REVOLUTION OR EVOLUTION?

OLE D MADSEN

Introduction: the beta-cell and diabetes

As something relatively new, one can today permit oneself to say that an insulin deficit is the common denominator for all types of diabetes. The beta-cell is a highly specialized and therefore unique type of cell, the only cell in the body that has the property of being able to 'exploit' or read the insulin gene with formidable effectiveness. The beta-cell is the body's only source of the vital hormone, insulin. The autoimmune destruction of beta-cells in type 1 diabetes (T1D), and the ensuing absolute lack of insulin result in a lifelong course of treatment with daily insulin injections. Type 2 diabetes (T2D) with peripheral insulin resistance poses enormous demands for a surplus production of insulin that the existing beta-cells cannot meet. It is thus a matter of an absolute versus a relative lack of insulin and thereby of functional beta-cells in T1D versus T2D. The beta-cell has been accorded star status in diabetes research – and it is apparent that if it proves possible to re-establish a suitable quantity of functional beta-cells, it will also be possible to cure diabetes. Research projects that seek to translate basic developmental biological knowledge into the controlled maturing of stem cells into beta-cells have thus been one of the main activities at Hagedorn Research Institute (HRI) for a number of years. The institute is centrally placed in internationally cutting-edge consortiums with the mission of developing cell-mediated therapy of diabetes based on stem cells and regeneration.

The background – the Hagedorn Research Laboratorium and 64K – the GAD story

The following sections give an account of my own story seen in the light of beta-cell research. This is a story that reflects many aspects of the unique workplaces that the University of Chicago, the Hagedorn Research Institute and Steno Diabetes Center have been over the years. In retrospect, mine may seem to have been a well-planned career with a clear focus on cell therapy. In reality, things were strikingly different – the product of a mixture of chance events, curiosity, freedom of action and of the fact that it was the period's most important basic immunological questions that set the real agenda. My first acquaintanceship with Hagedorn Research Laboratorium was thus a one-day visit (as a science student) to research chiefs Bruno Hansen and Åke Lernmark in 1980. The laboratory had been detached from Steno just a few years earlier, where it had functioned as the hospital's research laboratory for a period of more than 20 years. Although it was now an independent research laboratory with its own management, the umbilical cord to Steno was never entirely severed, since Nerup, Deckert and Binder retained their research groups at Hagedorn. SDC's presence has to date remained an integral part of HRI. Åke's research focus was the immunological cause of T1D – strongly inspired by Nerup's pioneering work on the HLA association. And with Steinunn Bækkeskov and Åke's demonstration of beta-cell surface autoantibodies in T1D patients – directed at "64K" (*Nature* 1982) – their energy was now focused on finding the antigen on the beta-cell's surface that might be the direct cause of diabetes. Bruno Hansen was an insulin chemist and at the same time head of R&D at Nordisk Gentofte. In that role, Bruno was deeply involved in the production of recombinant human insulin.

For Åke, the goal was clear: monoclonal antibodies against the beta-cell specific autoantigen were to ensure the final identification, so the gene could be cloned – and thereby become the key to recombinant antigen production and vaccination against diabetes.

In addition to discussing a possible future in Chicago, I was introduced to the method by which one isolates islets of Langerhans. This may sound banal, but it was and is an important component of the backbone in many research projects at both Hagedorn and Steno – and part of the glue that indissolubly linked the two institutions. Thus, the islet-fishing students have always existed – in one department – first under Jens Høiriis Nielsen's and Hanne Richter Olesen's legendary leadership – and today under Allan Karlsen and Tina Olsen, Novo Nordisk in Måløv, but with the activities still taking place at Hagedorn. The "64K protein" remained pivotal in Åke's and Steinunn's work, also after they left Hagedorn (Åke for a professorship in Seattle in 1988/89 – and Steinunn for University of California at San Francisco in 1990/91). With steady islet deliveries from Hagedorn to Steinunn at UCSF, an astonishing breakthrough took place with the demonstration of "64K" as a cytoplasmatic enzyme: glutamic acid decarboxylase (GAD) – and thus not a surface protein. The cloning race was on. Birgitte Michelsen (the head of Hagedorn's molecular biological laboratory) and Allan Karlsen (who went with Åke to Seattle) each cloned a mammal isoform of GAD (67K and 65K respectively). With uncannily good timing, both works were published in the same issue of PNAS, with Don Steiner communicating both articles to the journal. Continued work on the development of assays for the detection of anti-GAD antibodies later led to the discovery that these antibodies can also be demonstrated in T2D patients who slowly 'convert' from T2D to T1D (known as LADA or Latent Autoimmune Diabetes in Adults).

Bruno Hansen's work in Nordisk Gentofte R&D, in collaboration with Rutter & Bell, Chiron and UCSF, led to an effective process for the production of recombinant human insulin. Bruno left HRI relatively soon after the merger between Novo and Nordisk Gentofte. Jørn Nerup was therefore acting head of research in the interim period (1990/91) until the appointment of Pierre De Meyts.

The Don Steiner Lab, University of Chicago – 1981-83

A combination of fascination with immunology, the infinite antibody repertoire obtained by the use/recycling of a limited gene material, my introduction into the hybridoma technology and production of monoclonal antibodies at the University of Aarhus along with my crucial brief meeting with Åke Lernmark in 1980 at Hagedorn resulted in my appointment immediately after my finals in the summer of 1981 as 'postdoc' at the University of Chicago under Professor Donald F. Steiner, the discoverer of proinsulin. This was my introduction to some incredibly fascinating diabetes research and to an environment where the biggest names in the field came on visits and set their mark on our everyday work. Åke often came by – with his splendid, contagious commitment and updated us on "64K". Don Steiner remained a lifelong mentor and source of inspiration.

Projects directed at the identification of diabetes-related autoantibodies with the help of hybridoma techniques led, among other things, to the production of C-peptide and proinsulin-specific monoclonal antibodies. These antibodies would later prove to be invaluable reagents, which both ended on the front page of the journal *Cell*, and also later secured me a permanent appointment at the Hagedorn Research Laboratory in 1985.

It was, however, my American colleague Allen Labrecques' allergy to laboratory rats that led to the first radical change in my research interests. The just finished race to clone the human insulin gene was to a certain extent conditioned by the fact that William Chick generated a transplantable x-ray-induced beta-cell tumour (insulinoma) in the local inbred strain of rats: the New England Diaconess Hospital Rat (NEDH rat) in Boston. Insulinoma propagation by transplantation competed with isolation of Langerhans islets as the source of the beta-cell material that later formed the basis for the isolation of rat insulin cDNA and the later cloning of the human gene [1]. Graeme Bell et al won this race [2], which was the fundamental step towards the present industrial production of recombinant human insulin and analogues of it. It was also a milepost that now inspired researchers to study the structure of the gene in order to understand its amazingly tissue-specific regulation.

The transplantable insulinoma and the derivation of multipotent endocrine stem cells

A routine delivery of tumour-bearing rats to the University of Chicago always comprised only one sex, and as the insulinoma was lethal within 2-3 weeks, the users of this tissue were completely dependent on the tumour propagation in Chick's laboratory. However, a pregnant tumour-bearing NEDH rat arrived and gave birth to its litter before the onset of lethal hypoglycaemia. With the help of a substitute mother, the offspring survived to form the basis of a local Chicago (and later Hagedorn) colony of the NEDH rat. This made possible a local transplantation activity that gave easy access to the much sought after insulinoma tissue. Among other things, the tissue was used in attempts at establishing *in vitro* cell cultures. Labrecques' severe allergy to experimental animals was the direct reason why I took over the project. In the first trial, I succeeded in establishing slow-growing cells with endocrine-like morphology. But the cells did not produce insulin. On transplantation to the NEDH rat, they now formed tumours that caused an unusually pronounced loss of weight and not the anticipated hypoglycaemic syndrome. We therefore became enthusiastic about these tumour cell cultures only when a re-test of media from cell cultivation trays with almost forgotten cultures from the cell incubator showed enormous quantities of insulin. This indicated the presence of multipotence, where insulin-producing variants could arise in long-term cultures. Cloning trials gave one single positive insulin-producing culture, which by virtue of the long doubling time had reached a number of cells that permitted seeding to a single 25 ml culture bottle – just before I left Don Steiner's laboratory to start at Hagedorn. With the cells in my breast pocket and an agreement with Åke for a key to the laboratory, I was thus able to ensure the continuance of this project by going straight from the airport to the incubators at Hagedorn.

The cells proved to be a goldmine able to keep me and a growing group of colleagues occupied for a number of years. In Lernmark's house, the enthusiastic and innovative project was provided with plenty of space – and the outcome proved to be the first well documented multipotent pancreatic endocrine stem cell (the MSL cell) that could develop and be preserved in different stages of hypoglycaemic insulinomas, anorectic glucagonomas and a somatostatinoma [3]. Over the years, many students have been involved in MSL cell studies, of whom Palle Serup, Helle Petersen, Jan Jensen and Mette Jørgensen have remained in basic pancreas research. Interactions with Jørn Nerup's group concerning the MSL cell will be described later.

Regulation of the insulin gene and developmental biology

The first steps towards acquiring more knowledge about the complex developmental biology that governs both the formation of the pancreas, and thereby that of the beta-cells, and also the stringent tissue-specific regulation of the insulin gene had been taken. The mentioned clonal studies required a clone-specific marker. From the USA, Jørn and Åke had headhunted the molecular biologist David Owerbach to Hagedorn, so we chose to use a 4-kilobase-long DNA fragment that David had cloned from his own white blood cells [4], and which contained a copy of the entire intact genomic, human insulin gene. We could now specifically follow the activation of the human insulin gene when the rat cell matured towards the beta-cell phenotype. When the beta-cell matured, both rat and human insulin were produced and released from these cells.

The insulin gene is the same in all our cells, and so of course are the promoter/enhancer sequences upstream to the coding sequence of the gene. Thus, the structure of the gene itself cannot explain why some genes are expressed only in special cells. The hunt now began to identify the transcription factors (proteins) that underlie the specificity.

Transcription factors – and the embryonic stem cell link to the renaissance of developmental biology

Many transcription factors that were able to recognize sequences in the insulin-enhancer/promoter structure were described. Some of these proteins proved to be relatively beta-cell specific. Helena Edlund's isolation of the IPF1 protein (later called the PDX1 protein), cloning of the IPF1 gene – and the generation of the null-mutation for IPF1/PDX1 in mice evoked attention in the scientific world, which was astonished to read in *Nature* that the mouse had no pancreas at all [5].

In 1981, embryonic stem cells (ES cells) in continuous cultures had been established in mice. They proved to be pluripotent, i.e. if these cells were injected back into a mouse blastocyst, they would enter into the formation of fully viable mice. The fact that it was possible to change the mouse's hereditary material with incredible precision in embryonic stem cells became the foundation for the renaissance of developmental biology.

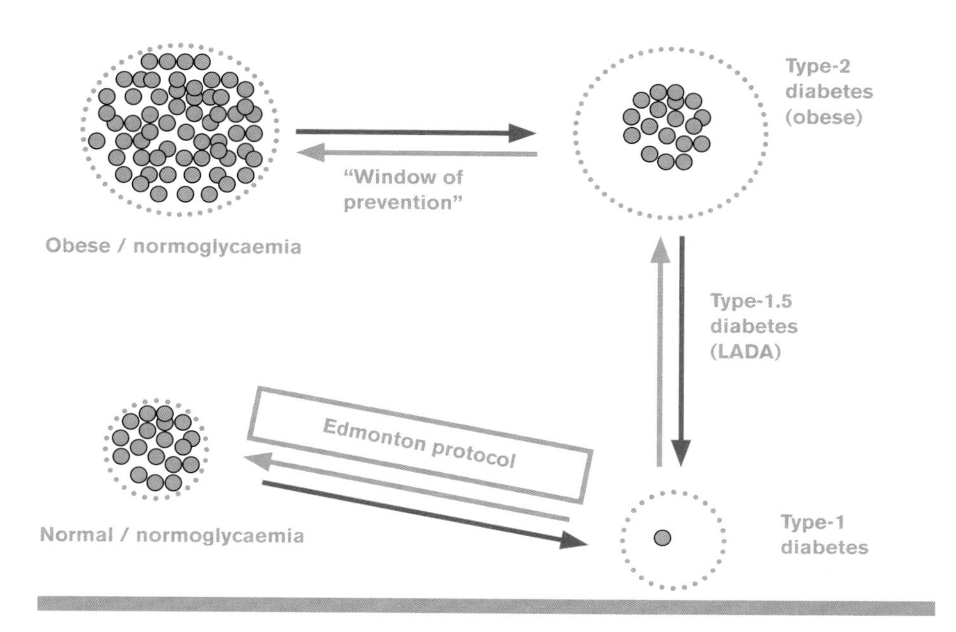

The beta-cell mass and diabetes. Fewer beta-cells (red arrows) lead to diabetes. Cell therapy and thereby reestablishment of a sufficiently functional beta-cell mass will normalize blood glucose control – and is thus a kind of cure for diabetes. (Data from the author).
LADA = Latent autoimmune diabetes in adults.

The astonishment at the total absence of a pancreas in Helena Edlund's PDX1 null-mutant was due to the view that PDX1 was a beta-cell specific (and insulin gene-specific) transcription factor [6]. It later became clear, however, that PDX1 was expressed in the entire duodenum and into the lower part of the stomach, but especially strongly in the pancreas under development. Thus, a child born without a pancreas proved to carry a homozygotic zero mutation in the human IPF1/PDX1-gene [7] – i.e. an identical phenotype in mouse and man. The developmental biology of the pancreas is incredibly well preserved through the evolution of the vertebrates – and the beta-cell is regarded as the 'oldest cell' or the founder of the pancreas itself [8].

The beta-cell carries an enormous responsibility: there must be no possibility of an insulin overdose, as severe hyperinsulinaemia will cause lethal hypoglycaemia. One can imagine a link between this fact and the presence of a uniquely heightened 'suicide preparedness' in the mature beta-cell (exemplified by the transplantable insulinoma's ability to eliminate the endogenous beta-cells [9]), which may in turn be an Achilles heel with a link to diabetes. Groundbreaking studies from Jørn Nerup's group show precisely that beta-cells have a unique vulnerability to cytokines, such as interleukin-1 and TNF-alpha [10, 11]. This vulnerability occurs selectively during beta-cell maturation, as shown through studies of multipotent MSL-cells – carried out in collaboration with Karin Nielsen, Allan Karlsen, Thomas Mandrup-Poulsen and Jørn Nerup.

The mature beta-cell and the early pancreatic stem cell

Today we know three transcription factors that are for the main part found selectively in beta-cells in connection with the mature pancreas. Besides PDX1, these are HlXB9 and NKX6.1. Common to all three is the fact that they are expressed in the earliest pancreatic rudiments and at the same time 2 of the 3 null-mutants have "global" pancreatic phenotypes with a total absence of a pancreas (PDX1) or of a dorsal pancreas (HlxB9).

It is therefore an obvious possibility that the phylogenetic developmental history is reflected in this ontogenetic pattern of expression, in which the beta-cell is regarded as the basis of the pancreatic phylogenesis. It may therefore be imagined that these early pancreatic stem cells have a primary potential for forming beta-cells – and that evolutionarily, moreover, they have at the same time acquired a developmental repertoire enabling them to form all types of pancreatic cells.

The laboratory's increasing interest in basic developmental biology, primarily driven by Jan Jensen and Palle Serup, resulted in pioneering analysis of the crucial importance of the Notch signalling for the development of the hormone-producing cells in the pancreas. Active Notch signalling is thus necessary to 'brake' or 'inhibit' the activation of endocrine cell maturation (which is governed by the transcription factor, Ngn3), in order at the same time to permit sufficient propagation of unspecialized, multipotent pancreatic stem cells (progenitor cells). Thus, in the absence of Notch signalling in the pancreas (exemplified in the Hes1 null-mutant), a premature upward regulation of Ngn3 takes place in the early pancreas rudiment, which leads to endocrine cell maturation (primarily glucagon-producing alpha-cells) – along with complete or partial depletion of the progenitor cells and thereby strong pancreatic hypoplasia [12].

Endocrine cells in the body have many features in common with neurons in the central nervous system. Pearse (Hammersmith Hospital, London) proposed the APUD (Amine Precursor Uptake and Decarboxylation) concept almost 40 years ago, which claimed that all endocrine cells came from migrant cells from *cresta neuralis* – i.e. that they were of ectodermal origin [13]. Even though classical studies indicate that both intestinal and pancreatic endocrine cells are of endodermal origin, it is possible as late as in 1982 to find this heading in *Nature*: *"Islet cell precursors are neurons"* [14]. As described by Skipper & Lewis in *Nature Genetics*, our Notch work has helped to open the understanding for a common regulation of the very parallel developmental patterns that in the endoderm versus the ectoderm lead to the formation of endocrine cells versus neurons [15]. Our Notch work was made possible by funding from the National Institutes of Health (NIH).

The Edmonton protocol: a kind of "proof of principle" for cell-based therapy of diabetes

As mentioned in the introduction, a re-establishment of a sufficient, functioning beta-cell mass could be predicted to be able to 'cure' diabetes. Groundbreaking studies in Edmonton by Shapiro et al show that intraportal infusion of donor islets of Langerhans to T1D patients can recreate a near-normal blood glucose regulation – without injection of insulin. However, one can by no means speak of a 'cure' for T1D, as the islets appear to die over time (~10 % are still insulin-free after 5 years) – in spite of continuous immune therapy. If near-normal blood glucose regulation can be recreated by cell-based therapy, the progression in the development of late-diabetic complications will probably be brought to a complete halt. A hunt for therapeutic beta-cells has therefore started and, as there is a lack of organ donors, the focus is naturally directed at stem cells.

The stem cell field has likewise exploded with a wealth of controversial articles claiming the presence of diverse potent stem cells that can be isolated from diverse organs. To cut a long story short, no data have so far been reproduced to support the claim that so-called 'adult' (or non-embryonic)

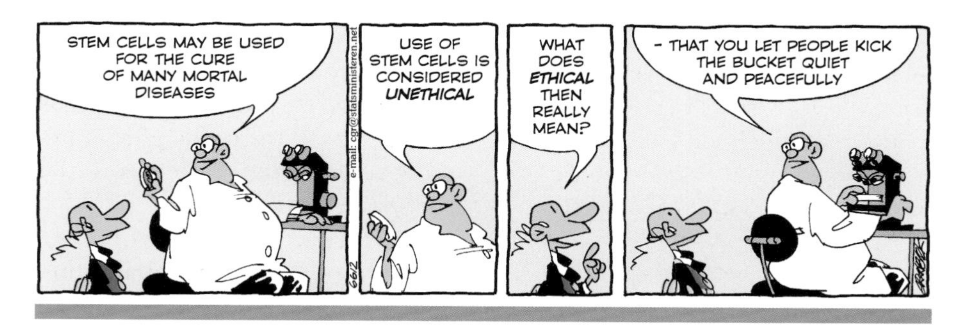

(Published with permission).

stem cells have the capacity to be used as the reliable and preferred source for generating therapeutic beta-cells.

That leaves the pluripotent embryonic stem cell. The laboratory at Hagedorn has reached a phase – primarily driven by Palle Serup – in which the goal is to try to translate the developmental biological knowledge into 'education' of ES cells *in vitro*, with the object of developing normal glucose-sensitive beta-cells.

This strategy has been stimulated by the Juvenile Diabetes Research Foundation (JDRF), which in collaboration with NIH has brought about the economic basis for the formation of the NIH-supported "*Beta Cell Biology Consortium*" (www.betacell.org). Since 2001, Hagedorn has been part of this consortium, where we both run a core function developing antibody reagents for the whole consortium and also head (Serup) an international research group working to obtain a deeper understanding of key processes in the beta-cell's development.

JDRF has also initiated the formation of "*JDRF-Center for Beta Cell Therapy in Diabetes*" – under the leadership of Daniel Pipeleers, Brussels (www.betacelltherapy.org). Hagedorn has been part of this centre since 2001, and we have now obtained EU support to generate therapeutic beta-cells from embryonic stem cells – again with a springboard in normal developmental biology.

Although this may appear unrealistically ambitious, the embryonic stem cell source is a possible key to a treatment that is comparable to an actual cure.

Perhaps this is wishful thinking – but if it can be done ..., it WILL be done.

REFERENCES

1. *Bell GI, Pictet RL, Rutter WJ, Cordell B, Tischer E, Goodman HM. Sequence of the human insulin gene. Nature 1980;284:26-32*
2. *Hall S. Invisible frontiers – the race to synthesize a human gene. New York: Oxford University Press, 1987:1-334*
3. *Madsen OD, Jensen J, Blume N, Petersen HV, Lund K, Karlsen C, Andersen FG, Jensen PB, Larsson LI, Serup P. Pancreatic development and matura-*

tion of the islet B cell. Studies of pluripotent islet cultures. Eur J Biochem 1996;242:435-45

4. *Owerbach D, Nerup J. Restriction fragment length polymorphism of the insulin gene in diabetes mellitus. Diabetes 1982;31: 275-7*
5. *Jonsson J, Carlsson L, Edlund T, Edlund H. Insulin-promoter-factor 1 is required for pancreas development in mice. Nature 1994;371:606-9*
6. *Petersen HV, Serup P, Leonard J, Michelsen BK, Madsen OD. Transcriptional regulation of the human insulin gene is dependent on the homeodomain protein STF1/IPF1 acting through the CT boxes. Proc Natl Acad Sci U S A 1994;91:10465-9*
7. *Stoffers DA, Zinkin NT, Stanojevic V, Clarke WL, Habener JE. Pancreatic agenesis attributable to a single nucleotide deletion in the human IPF1 gene coding sequence. Nat Genet 1997;15:106-10*
8. *Madsen OD. Pancreas phylogeny and ontogeny in relation to a 'pancreatic stem cell'. C R Biol 2007;330:534-7*
9. *Blume N, Skouv J, Larsson LI, Holst JJ, Madsen OD. Potent inhibitory effects of transplantable rat glucagonomas and insulinomas on the respective endogenous islet cells are associated with pancreatic apoptosis. J Clin Invest 1995;96:2227-35*
10. *Bendtzen K, Mandrup-Poulsen T, Nerup J, Nielsen JH, Dinarello CA, Svenson M. Cytotoxicity of human pI 7 interleukin-1 for pancreatic islets of Langerhans. Science 1986;232:1545-7*
11. *Mandrup-Poulsen T, Bendtzen K, Dinarello CA, Nerup J. Human tumor necrosis factor potentiates human interleukin 1-mediated rat pancreatic beta-cell cytotoxicity. J Immunol 1987;139:4077-82*
12. *Jensen J, Pedersen EE, Galante P, Hald J, Heller RS, Ishibashi M, Kageyama R, Guillemot F, Serup P, Madsen OD. Control of endodermal endocrine development by Hes-1. Nat Genet 2000;24:36-44*
13. *Pearse AG. The cytochemistry and ultrastructure of polypeptide hormone-producing cells of the APUD series and the embryologic, physiologic and pathologic implications of the concept. J Histochem Cytochem 1969;17:303-13*
14. *Pearse AG. Islet cell precursors are neurons. Nature 1982;295:96-7*
15. *Skipper M, Lewis J. Getting to the guts of enteroendocrine differentiation. Nat Genet 2000;24:3-4*

DANES, GREAT DANES, AND DIABETES – THE VIEW FROM ANOTHER COUNTRY

EDWIN AM GALE

> "You can tell a Dane anywhere, but you can't tell him (or her) anything"
>
> *Old English Proverb*

What have the Danes contributed to our understanding of diabetes? Or (as a Dane might express it), what haven't they contributed? My own relationship with the Danish people began 25 years ago, when, as a junior investigator, I had reached the stage at which I was expected to spend a year or two in the USA in order to obtain my BTA ("been to America") qualification. My boss and mentor at the time was Robert Tattersall, and I remember that we sat down together and discussed the options. All were impressive, none were appealing. Not long after, Robert returned from a visit to the Steno, and remarked in passing that the nurses were unusually attractive. There are certain defining moments in the life of a young investigator, and this was one of them. It was, little did I know it, to be the start of a long love affair with the Danish people in general, and with one Danish woman in particular.

Having declared this conflict of interest, as one is obliged to do these days, let me pass on to the main topic of this chapter. What have the Danes contributed to our understanding and treatment of diabetes? My answer will come in three parts. First, I will dwell on some of the great achievements of the past. Next, I will come to the present, and will ask why a small country like Denmark continues to make such a disproportionate contribution to diabetes? The answer, I believe, is to be found in the Danish character and culture, and my analysis of the Danish people, not entirely serious, will be found in the third and final section.

The Past

Insulin

Danish investigators were well known for their work in areas such as physiology and serum therapy, but appear to have paid little attention to diabetes before the advent of insulin. The work of August Krogh (1874–1949) on capillary function and gaseous exchange in tissues led to the award of the Nobel Prize for Physiology or Medicine in 1920. As a result he was invited to give a lecture tour in the USA and Canada in 1921, but the trip was delayed by family illness. Fatefully enough, his wife and long-time co-worker the physician and physiologist Birte Marie Jørgensen (known as Marie) had developed diabetes. Krogh recommended her to the care of Hans Christian Hagedorn (1888–1971), a rising young clinical investigator: Hagedorn had, as a country GP, developed a widely used method for the measurement of blood glucose with the aid of Norman Jensen, the local pharmacist. By 1921, Hagedorn was settled in Copenhagen and preparing to defend his thesis. Krogh's delayed visit to North America meant that he arrived at a time when the medical world was resonating with the discovery of insulin. There followed a meeting with Macleod in Toronto, and the Kroghs sailed back to Europe with the licence to manufacture insulin in Scandinavia. Hagedorn was the natural partner in this work, and the two worked together so effectively that they produced a pancreatic extract that could throw a rabbit into hypoglycaemic convulsions within nine days of Krogh's disembarkation in Copenhagen. This story has been related so well by Torsten Deckert [1] that we need dwell on only a few of its features.

Hagedorn was a heavily built and impressive man, at times both brave and honest when it was politic not to be (for example during the German occupation), but also somewhat remote: he was generally referred to by his initials. He was imperious, at times uncontrollably irascible, and by no means easy company. This soon led to a row with two of his senior employees, the Pedersen brothers, with the result that they went off to found a new insulin company, appropriately called Novo, in 1925. This was not the only time that Hagedorn's temper worked to his disadvantage. Despite these altercations, the business boomed. Nordisk insulin was exported with great success because of its reputation for quality. A spoiling campaign launched by the British insulin manufacturers, based around the pious claim that pork insulin was offensive to the sensibilities of Jewish people with diabetes, fooled no-one [1].

Meanwhile painstaking chemical analysis by JJ Abel and his team had by 1926 resulted in the preparation of insulin in a form so pure that it could be crystallised – the first protein for which this was possible. It was assumed at the time that crystallisation guaranteed the absolute purity of the preparation, but later experience showed this to be untrue, and early insulins contained a horrendous mix of other biological material. This included potent digestive enzymes which work best in the alkaline juice secreted by the pancreas, and are rendered inactive by acid. These enzymes were slowly eliminated, but for forty years most insulins were prepared in acid solution, which had the further advantage of improving the solubility of insulin and any stray foreign proteins that might be present. Insulin treatment was always, as Maurice Chevalier said of old age, to be preferred to the alternative, but such preparations frequently caused unpleasant allergic reactions, sometimes swelling to angry lumps half the size of an orange following each injection.

Improved purity had some effect on the frequency of these side-effects, but also meant that insulin was more quickly absorbed, and therefore more rapidly washed out of the system. Blood glucose fell with each injection but bounced back up again after 3-4 hours as its effect wore off. In the 1930s Michael Somogyi demonstrated in St Louis that stable control could be achieved with four daily injections, one before each meal, and one at 3 am! A long-acting insulin was clearly needed, but none existed at the time.

A wide range of additives was tried before Hagedorn thought of adding an alkaline protein in the attempt to render insulin more soluble at a neutral pH. Norman Jensen, his faithful assistant, pointed out that few proteins are in fact alkaline. Among these was protamine, a low molecular weight protein found in sperm. A series of experiments showed that protamine could indeed form a complex with insulin and prolong its action for 12 hours or more. Fish have extravagant sexual habits, and are therefore well-endowed with sperm; it later emerged that protamine is unusually well tolerated by the immune system and that allergic reactions are incredibly rare. Adding protamine did of course raise the pH of the insulin to which it was added, making it less stable, and this could at first only be overcome by preparing it in an acid solution for storage and instructing the patient to inject a measured amount of buffer into the vial to neutralise the solution before use.

It took another ten years before Nordisk chemists found that a stable neutral solution could be obtained by mixing soluble insulin with protamine in isophane (precisely balanced) proportions with the correctly judged amount of zinc and preservatives. This became known to millions as NPH (neutral protamine Hagedorn) or isophane insulin. Joslin was so impressed that he named an era in diabetes management in honour of the achievement. The earliest era (1898-1914) was named in honour of the German physician Naunyn, the next (1914-1922) was the Allen era, named for Frank Allen whose starvation regimen prolonged the lives, but all too often merely extended the suffering, of children with diabetes. The subsequent era

(1922–1936) was named for Banting, and the period between January 1 1937 and December 31 1943 became the Hagedorn era [2].

In a strange sad echo of events in Toronto, the achievement seems to have brought little personal happiness to those involved. When it became necessary to take out a patent on protamine insulin, Hagedorn unreasonably insisted that the patent should be in the name of his laboratory assistant and companion Lise Wodstrup. Norman Jensen was particularly vulnerable because their working arrangements were informal, and the ensuing rift between Hagedorn and himself was bitter and for always. Formal resolution was reached when Hagedorn, Wodstrup and Jensen vested their rights in the company, with the arrangement that profits should be channelled into a new charitable trust. Jensen was packed off with a cheque – a paltry amount in terms of the profit that was later to be made from NPH insulin, although this was scarcely dreamed of at the time. Hagedorn never buried the hatchet on any grievance, and his war with the Pedersen brothers now entered a new and even more bitter phase. Insulin manufacturers had to be able to make the new insulin, but the basic step in formulation belonged to Nordisk. Thus it was that Hagedorn claimed that his patent had been infringed when Novo made *Protamine Zinc Insulin*; the result was an ugly legal battle.

The outcome, as always, was messy, and the hostility between the two organizations persisted well into the 1980s. One positive result of the feud was that Novo persisted in the hunt for another means of prolonging the action of insulin, and Knud Hallas-Møller finally hit upon one in 1944 during the Nazi occupation of Denmark, although further years of development were to be needed before it reached commercial production. The principle was addition of extra zinc to a neutral insulin solution, plus special seeding techniques that created crystals of varying size that dissolved very slowly after injection. These were the zinc or *Lente®* insulins, and much effort went into developing the best mix of small and large crystals to make a once daily insulin. And there it rested. Despite endless attempts, no better means of retarding the action of insulin other than protamine or zinc could be found until genetically modified insulins became available 50 years later. Danish insulins ruled the world.

Another small observation was to hold great importance for the future of insulin treatment. World War 2 caused rationing of insulin in all the Scandinavian countries, and patient registers were therefore needed. In Sweden this impressed upon a physician called Jorpes the high frequency of allergic reactions to insulin. It happened that a patient came to see him one day with very distressing allergic problems. By chance he had some ultrapure insulin sitting on his desk; he had prepared this for a laboratory experiment by means of repeated crystallisation. On impulse he made up a solution, treated the patient with it, and solved her problems. This showed beyond question that insulin allergy was due to residual impurities in the preparation, and the quest for ultra-pure insulins was launched, actively espoused by Jorgen Schlichtkrull of Novo, whose daughter suffered from unstable diabetes. Locked into their fraternal feud, the Danish manufacturers were to lead the way into a new era of insulin therapy.

The Present

Diabetes research in Denmark

Underpinned by the success of the insulin manufacturers, and the support this generated for patient care and research, Danish diabetes entered a new era in the second half of the twentieth century. Jacob Poulsen (1907-1988), one of nature's gentlemen and a wonderful raconteur, launched a research tradition at the Steno and founded what was to become the Hagedorn Research Institute in 1957. Knud Lundbæk (1912-1995) was another of the great figures of Danish diabetes. His long and distinguished career passed through three stages: first as a surrealist poet in Paris, next as an eminent diabetologist (1943-79), and finally as a noted expert on China. His intellectual capacity was such that he began the formal study of classical Chinese at the age of 70, and became a noted expert in the field. His landmark work on long term diabetes, published in 1953, brought the toll of diabetic complications into sharp focus, and Lundbæk's interest in the relationship between the anterior hypophysis, growth hormone and diabetic retinopathy promoted a new phase in research, as well as practice of ablating the pituitary in the often unsucessful attempt to prevent blindness. His influence on a generation of diabetes doctors was immense, and his sardonic humour is still remembered. For example, in 1985 he attended the first Knud Lundbæk Lecture of the Scandinavian Society for the Study of Diabetes with the comment that "*it was a strange feeling to sit there and it occurred to me that it would have been more proper for me to be dead than to be alive on such an occasion*" [3].

Danish research in diabetes has always been notable for its clinical focus, its emphasis on the physiological basis of disease, and its ability to maintain a sustained focus upon chosen areas of research over decades of painstaking endeavour. Take, for example, the kidney. Torsten Deckert and Jacob Poulsen published a follow-up survey of 307 patients diagnosed under the age of 31 before 1933; the 10-year mortality was 20 % in those from remoter country areas, and one third of the remainder went on to develop diabetic nephropathy [4]. This was to change. Carl Erik Mogensen had already noted that anti-hypertensive therapy reduced the rate of protein excretion in diabetic kidney disease [5], and Hans-Henrik Parving went on to establish that early aggressive anti-hypertensive therapy could greatly slow progression of diabetic nephropathy [6]; observations that – backed by his towering presence and emphatic presentation – resulted in changes of management that offered years of freedom from dialysis and extended life for many people with diabetes around the world. And this was just the beginning, for further studies by Danish investigators have led the world in clarifying the genetics, physiology, pathology and treatment of diabetic kidney disease.

This chapter does not set out to catalogue the many achievements of the past and present generation of talented diabetes investigators in Denmark, but special mention must be made of the role of Jørn Nerup in uncovering the autoimmune basis of juvenile-onset (later type 1) diabetes. His thesis work on Addison's clarified the existence of tubercular and idiopathic forms of the disease, and the latter, as also noted by previous investigators, overlapped with juvenile diabetes. Early investigations suggested a role for cellular immunity in the pathogenesis of diabetes, and this was followed by the first report of its HLA associations [7].

There are those chroniclers of science who argue endlessly about "who did what first?". These, in my experience, have little insight into the way science advances. Did you know, for instance, that the websites of three diabetes research units in the USA lay claim to the synthesis of the insulin gene? All three are wrong, for diabetes researchers at the three institutions had nothing whatsoever to do with it [8]. It all goes to show that, as George Orwell pointed out in *1984*, he who controls the present also controls the past, or – as my father told me long ago – you can achieve almost anything you want in your professional career, just so long as you don't also want to get the credit for having done it. Nerup will be remembered for the priority he gained in making some landmark observations, but his more lasting achievement has been the sustained research and development that he guided or stimulated over the following decades, research that opened doors into the cellular basis of immunity, the role of cytokines, genetic analysis and clinical intervention studies. This stamina and persistence, let me repeat, is one of the hallmarks of Danish research into diabetes.

The Danish character

If you offer praise to a Dane, you are guaranteed to secure his or her attention. The Danes are indeed well-equipped to fight their own battles, and they do not submit gracefully. I learned this in 1981 as I began my long and largely unsuccessful struggle to master the Danish language. Danish has no fewer than 8 vowels, three of which were designed without reference to the anatomy and function of the human vocal chords. Add to this that correct Danish (*rigsdansk*) makes major use of the glottal stop (a totally redundant apposition of the vocal chords in the middle of a vowel, resulting in the sort of sound you might make when swallowing a frog), and it is easy to forget that English is in fact a Danish dialect. This family relationship becomes obvious when you compare the written forms of the two languages, the main difference being that the English, benefiting from their numerous invaders, also borrowed a range of French words to express a number of important abstract concepts which the Danes never got round to formulating.

But I digress. The point is that I learned a lot about the Danish character when I attempted to improve my language skills by reading a Danish account of the Battle of Copenhagen. Briefly, this battle, fought on April 2nd 1801, went as follows. The British fleet lay to the north of Copenhagen, and the Danish fleet was anchored along the shoreline of the city, supported by numerous floating gun platforms. The key to the Danish position was the island of Trekroner, which formed the northern end of the Danish battle line; the heavy guns mounted on this fortified island were guaranteed to pound the enemy ships to pieces as they sailed past to engage the Danish fleet. Confounding expectation, Nelson, the junior British Admiral, took his squadron over the shoals of the outer passage between Amager and the island of Saltholm to engage the Danish fleet from the less defended southern end of the line. The British ships were bigger, and manned by battle-hardened sailors, so the ferocity of the defence came as a surprise and resulted in a thousand British casualties. In the midst of all this confusion, Nelson's commander hoisted the signal instructing Nelson to retreat. Raising his telescope to his blind eye, Nelson exclaimed that *"I really do not see the signal!"* The battle ended when the entire Danish fleet had surrendered or been disabled, and the city of Copenhagen had agreed to a flag of truce. With some justice, the British regard this as one of their more crushing naval victories, so I was surprised to find that the chapter following this description began with a question. The question was: "*Who won?*". I had yet to learn that the Danes are a stubborn people.

More seriously, one has to ask how it is that a country the size of Denmark has made such an exceptional contribution to our knowledge of diabetes. One reason, as already mentioned, has been the success of the insulin manufacturers, coupled with the determination of Hagedorn and the other pioneers to channel the dividends of their work into research and patient care. The consequence has been a healthy interaction and exchange of personnel between the academic and pharmaceutical research sectors. Another factor has been the intensity of the competition for academic posts, ensuring that only the most energetic and talented have risen to the post of chief physician. Once in post, however, such individuals have obtained the security and support needed to plan and direct very long term programmes of research. This, as already emphasised, has allowed Danish research to sustain its focus upon a few selected areas of genuine clinical importance.

There is of course a down side to all this. The power and influence of the chief physicians has been such that basic scientists have sometimes felt frustrated in their careers. Given the importance of basic science, we can expect that a fairer balance between basic and clinical science will emerge, but my own hope is that Danish researchers will remain light on their feet. By this I mean that they should value their outstanding ability to identify soluble problems related to clinical care, and should where possible avoid the scaled-up production line strategy needed to compete successfully in some areas of molecular biology.

Another obvious strength of diabetes research in Denmark has been its ability to attract an almost endless supply of talented and highly motivated young investigators. Non-Danes may not appreciate this, but Danes don't like to travel. Few, if any, of their leading investigators have spent any time working abroad, and you will rarely find a young Dane among the army of young overseas research fellows in American institutions. Why should this be? Danes just prefer to stay in Denmark. If you don't understand why this should be, ask a young investigator from Scotland why he or she prefers not to work in England, and you will be on your way to an answer. Denmark is a flat country, but when you are there the rest of the world just seems to be downhill.

What becomes of all these bright young people? I often used to wonder. There is not enough room for them in the upper echelons of diabetes research, but the research training acquired at institutions such as the Steno opens the door to careers in many other clinical specialities, while others move into the pharmaceutical industry. Elsewhere in the world, the clinical pathway rapidly clogs with people who cannot move onwards and upwards, but Denmark does seem to have solved the problem. Let us hope that the administrators never set out to rationalise the situation.

Last, but not least, we come on to the patients. Here we touch once again upon a vital feature of the Danish character. The Danes are remarkable for their ability to be very liberal yet very conservative at one and the same time. There are many examples of their liberalism. They were, for example, the first country in Europe to decide that it is legal to have sex with animals[1]. Contrast this with my own country, where such an activity carried

---

1 I must hasten to dispel the mischievous rumour that Danish law requires signed consent from both participants, although this did give rise to a string of unconvincing forgeries, many originating from the region around Århus.

a sentence of life imprisonment until very recently. More notably, the Nazi round-up of the Jewish population of Denmark, planned for October 1st 1943, was forestalled by *"an extraordinary operation involving the whole Danish people and the agreement of the Swedish government, nearly all Danish Jews were hidden and then ferried across to Sweden"* [9]. As for the conservative aspect, it must be said that the Danes are remarkably compliant people. Even their hippies wear uniform. And they come second only to the British in their ability to radiate silent disapproval. The visitor to Copenhagen soon learns, for example, that it is not wise to cross the street when the little red man is illuminated, never mind the absence of any vehicles. It is better to wait with all the others. This willingness to comply, to my mind, arises from an unusually strong sense of shared identity. From our present point of view, however, this sense of hidden rules and shared identity translates into an extraordinary willingness to participate in research studies. There is, in conclusion, something very Danish about diabetes research in Denmark.

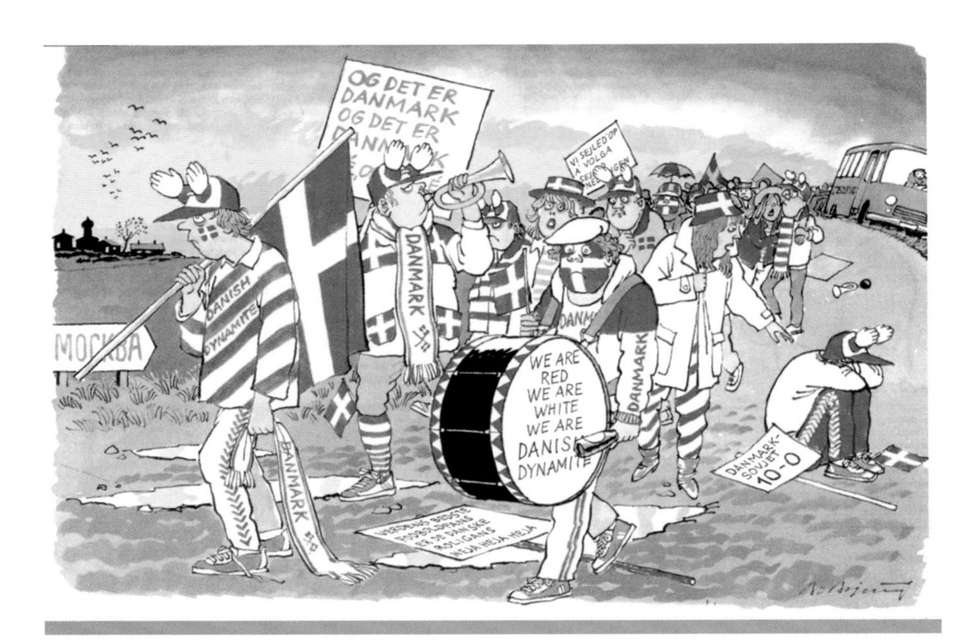

(Published with permission).

REFERENCES

1. *Deckert T. H.C.Hagedorn and Danish Insulin. Herning, Denmark: The Poul Christensen Publishing Co, 2000*
2. *Poulsen JE. Features of the History of Diabetology. Copenhagen: Munksgaard, 1982*
3. *Mungello DE. Knud Lundbaek (1912-1995). J Asian Stud 1995;54:921-3*
4. *Deckert T, Poulsen JE, Larsen M. Prognosis of diabetics with diabetes onset before the age of thirty-one. I. Survival, causes of death, and complications. Diabetologia 1978;14:363-70*
5. *Mogensen CE. Progression of nephropathy in long-term diabetics with proteinuria and effect of initial anti-hypertensive treatment. Scand J Clin Lab Invest 1976;36:383-8*
6. *Parving H-H, Andersen AR, Smidt UM, Svendsen PA. Early aggressive antihypertensive treatment reduces rate of decline in kidney function in diabetic nephropathy. Lancet 1983;i:1175-9*
7. *Nerup J, Platz P, Anderson OO, Christy M, Lyngsoe J, Poulsen JE, Ryder LP, Nielsen JS, Thomsen M, Svejgaard A. HL-A antigens and diabetes mellitus. Lancet 1974;ii:864-6*
8. *Hall SS. Invisible Frontiers. The Race to Synthesise a Human Gene. Tempus, 1987*
9. *Dawidowicz L. The War against the Jews 1933-45. Penguin Books, 1975*

AUTHORS

Ole Ortved Andersen, DMSc, ortvedandersen@mail.dk

Henning Beck-Nielsen, Professor, DMSc, henning.beck-nielsen@ouh.regionsyddanmark.dk

Christian Binder, DMSc, cbi@steno.dk

Knut Borch-Johnsen, Professor, DMSc, kbjo@steno.dk

Jens Sandahl Christiansen, Professor, DMSc, jsc@ki.au.dk

Torsten Deckert, DMSc, torsten.deckert@sol.dk

Bo Feldt-Rasmussen, Senior Lecturer, DMSc, bfr@rh.dk

Allan Flyvbjerg, Professor, DMSc, allan.flyvbjerg@dadlnet.dk

Edwin Gale, Professor, DMSc, edwin.gale@bristol.ac.uk

Jens Juul Holst, Professor, DMSc, holst@mfi.ku.dk

Klavs Jørgensen, Civil Engineer, klavs@post7.tele.dk

Claus Kühl, DMSc, ckuhl@kowaus.com

Torsten Lauritzen, Professor, DMSc, tl@alm.au.dk

Sten Madsbad, Professor, DMSc, sten.madsbad@hvh.regionh.dk

Ole Madsen, Professor, PhD, odm@hagedorn.dk

Thomas Mandrup-Poulsen, Professor, DMSc, tmpo@steno.dk

Carl Erik Mogensen, Professor, DMSc, carl.erik.mogensen@ki.au.dk

Lars Mølsted-Pedersen, DMSc, molsted.p@mail.dk

Jørn Nerup, Professor, DMSc, jne@steno.dk

Oluf Borbye Pedersen, Professor, DMSc, oluf@steno.dk

Flemming Pociot, Professor, DMSc, fpoc@steno.dk

Helle Terkildsen, RN, PhD-student, htm@alm.au.dk

Hans Ørskov, Professor, DMSc, hans.orskov@ki.au.dk